FORWARD Copyright © 2023 by Kellye Jones. All

rights reserved.

Printed in the United States of America. No part of this book may be used or reproduced in any manner whatsoever without written permission except in the case of brief quotations embodied in critical articles and reviews. For more information, contact Kellye Jones, c/o 2continueforward@gmail.com.

Inspiration for Writing the Book

Going from being misunderstood to being considered a genius or being told, "You don't know anything because you do not have a PhD." To "You have to be one of the smartest people I know." is something I experienced daily, in new circles, as an adult. This continued until I went back to the fundamentals I learned about communication as an adolescent.

As an only child, I had to discuss my day, three times a day every weekday, with my parents: my mother at 4:00 pm after school; my parents during dinner at 6:30 pm; and then my dad at 8:00 pm during our five-mile walk. During these conversations, I became very grounded in truth, transparency, context, and application.

Over the years, I mastered how to engage, educate, excite, and empower a crowd. My senior year in high school, I won my senior class superlative "Most Talkative". My senior year in college, I was the first undergraduate Teacher's Assistant for a Communications college course on legal ethics. Today, I am a life coach who helps people use their strengths and preferred communication style to maximize their fulfillment.

Recently, the DSM-5 added Social Pragmatic Communication Disorder (SPCD) to its list of diagnosable mental health conditions. This diagnosis is rooted in a person's misunderstanding of context and social understandings. Conversely, when people understand and firmly believe in their unique strengths, they able to more positively, effectively, confidently, and concisely (verbally and nonverbally) communicate their thoughts. This opens the doors for greater inner peace, depth, and fun.

This book, FORWARD – It is Tangible, equips readers with pathways to navigate towards greater joy. They will unmask their character strengths, master communication effectiveness, and obtain more fulfillment with future goal completions.

Let's talk about strengths. Let's talk about achieving your dreams.

To my students, teachers, physicians, ministers, and peers: you've got this.

I have heard your simple request to be heard and understood, and I have listened to your concerns about gaps and voids in communication, societal expectations, and as-yet unfulfilled dreams.

This book provides content that will enable you to bring your A-game to every social setting. The tools provided will ensure you are engaged, having fun, and feeling more fulfilled in your daily activities.

Let's go. Let's go!

Preface

Psychologist Valentina M. Pacheco-Cornejo and I are the volunteer cohosts of *The Moving Forward Podcast – Stories of Triumph*. We interview guests who have overcome mental health and physical challenges such as concussions, aneurysms, eyelid cancer, and more. Our guests have overcome bullying, domestic violence, suicidal ideations, grief, and more.

Our goal is to help listeners discover more pathways to move forward. Whether battling a potentially fatal condition or chronic mental health challenges, our guests mention their many failed attempts to get much-needed help. Our guests have faced roadblocks in conveying the urgency, duration, and frequency of their pain to their care providers. These roadblocks led them to over-generalized diagnoses, missed diagnoses, and misdiagnoses.

Even though, our guests had medical results such as MRIs, concussions, a noted withdrawal from social activities, and visible expressions of pain; their concerns were overlooked by those in whom they confided. As a result of their determination and confidence in their increasingly effective, concise communication skills, they did not stop telling their stories until they found someone who understood them. They had to go beyond passive listening and nodding of heads to unearth audiences with empathy and fortitude.

The great self- reporting and persistence of our podcast guests led to them and/or their family members finding persons who understood their hope and actively supported their desire for better health. There were periods of exhaustion, doubts, fear, and extended pauses to regroup along their journeys. They and their loved ones are now moving forward with stories of hope and triumph.

Pause when you need the respite, but don't stop. Your story of discovery and triumph will build you and many others up. You are

> You may encounter many defeats, but you must not be defeated. In fact, it may be necessary to encounter the defeats, so you can know who you are, what you can rise from, how you can still come out of it. -- Maya Angelou

Table of CONTENTS

Inspiration for Writing the Book 4
Dedication 6
Preface 8
Foreword 12
Acknowledgments and Thanks 14
Introduction 16
Chapter One: Introspective 18
    Whose Expectations? 22
    Deconstructing Thoughts 24
    Cognitive Flexibility 25
Chapter Two: Communication Strengthening 26
Chapter Three: Mindset 30
Chapter Four: Self-Assessment 36
    Self–Assessment of Transparency and Strengths-Based Goal Analysis
.... 38
Chapter Five: Edge- Unmask Your Greatness 50
    Myer's Briggs 53
Chapter Six: Sidelined- I Never Had the Whole Picture 58
    It's Time to Fill in the Gap 58
    Task Analysis 64
Chapter Seven: Who I Enjoy 68
    Positive Psychology's 24 Character Strengths 70
Chapter Eight: What I Think 72
    Stuck – Societal Expectations 74
    Conformation Bias 75
    Psychoneuroimmunology 76
    Doctor's Visit 79
Chapter Nine: When Time Management and Availability 88
    Availability 91
Chapter Ten: Where I Am Ready to Go 94
    Social Settings and Personality Types 99
    Social Behaviors 100

Ambiverts	101
Introverts	102
Extroverts	103
Omniverts	104
Chapter Eleven: Why -The Big Picture	106
Let's Learn More about Your Personality Strengths	108
The Big Five Assessment	109
The HEXACO Personality Inventory Assessment	118
Chapter Twelve: How - The Details	120
Chapter Thirteen: "Why" People and "How" People	122
Chapter Fourteen: VARK and Multi-Intellectual	128
Chapter Fifteen: Assess, Advance, and Stay Agile	132
The Five Love Languages	134
Advanced Self-Care	136
Wheel of Life's Self-Care Assessment	138
Chapter Sixteen: Constructive and Motivational Feedback	144
Chapter Seventeen: Making Your Next Move Forward	146
Achieve It with HEART	152
HEART by Kellye Jones	154
Chapter Eighteen: Get it!	158
Chapter Nineteen: Pay it Forward	162
About The Author	164
Glossary	170
References	176

Foreword

Often, I hear people discuss the weight of not living up to societal expectations. Sometimes we get so caught up in everything else that we forget our dreams and feel empty.

If you are not pursuing your dreams using your unique gifts, talents, and interests at least every once in a while, you may begin to undervalue *yourself*.

Life is full of opportunities to understand what you want and to get busy going after it.

Making time to dig deeper in understanding what makes you happiest, will bring forth more engaging encounters, stronger relationships, and fun.

You deserve more fulfillment. You got this.

Let's go. Let's go!

Acknowledgments and Thanks

In memory of my parents, **Walter Jones and Shelve Jones**: I love you, Mommy and Daddy. You provided the foundation for excellence with an emphasis on diversity and pivoting. I am becoming because you became.

Blaike Bibbs, Jay Bibbs, and Noah Bibbs: You are my gifts from God. You are my inspiration and my joy. I love you so much.

Certified Life Coach Institute: Thank you for your continued availability and support of my Life Coaching career. https://forwardlifecoach.com

Delta Sigma Theta Sorority, Inc: Thank you for your resilience, commitment, patience, guidance, and Sisterhood. I know I am never alone.

Introduction

One of my favorite childhood stories is "The Ugly Duckling." A mother duck hatches multiple eggs. One of her ducklings looks, quacks, and waddles differently from its siblings. The duckling tries extremely hard to fit in but always seems to miss the mark. After being ostracized and ridiculed, the duck runs away from home. The following year, the duck admires the beauty of a group of swans gliding across a lake. After reflecting on his year of never being enough, his head sinks low. This action makes him view his own reflection in the lake.

Immediately he realizes he is not a duck. He is a beautiful swan. He then proudly swims out of his isolation to swim with the swans. He finally understands his strength.

FORWARD It is Tangible provides tools to customize a strategic plan to greater fulfillment. Imagine fewer people masking, camouflaging, and experiencing micro stressors in their lives. There are endless possibilities for collaboration, support, influence, and success when you know your fierceness.

Let's move beyond the limiting societal expectations of onlookers and boredom. It's time to get excited about you and all of your awesomeness.

Success is tangible. FORWARD is Tangible. Fulfillment is accessible and tangible.

> We need quiet time to examine ourselves openly and honesty- spending quiet time alone gives your mind an opportunity to renew itself and create order. -- Susan Taylor

Chapter One:
Introspective

Pick a typical day to take your first assessments. Use these results as a baseline for your strengths, interests, and goals. They will be your point of comparison for progress. As time passes, you can look back at them and say, "I am making progress." or "I was not fulfilled because I was following someone else's dream. Now I understand my dream and I am moving FORWARD with intentionality." Try to include as many details as possible. Write in pen and feel free to use cross outs with a line over a word but do not completely delete anything you write.

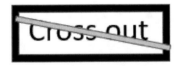

Items can be added or crossed out daily. Crossing out and keeping previous thoughts will enable you to find them quickly if you change your mind. It will help to track how your skills can be used to help you meet your goals. You will know what alliances and supports you must develop to achieve your dreams.

Keep in mind there is a difference between enablers and alliances. Enablers who do the work for you can stunt self-confidence and deflate self-advocacy. Enablers will complete a task using their frame of reference/ historical data. If the goal is your dream, and you want it to reflect your authentic self, you have to stay active in the process.

Alliances will do the work with you, short-term or long-term. The goal is to allow you both to keep excelling in your communication skills and overall gifts as you work toward task completion.

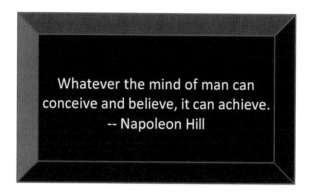

Whatever the mind of man can conceive and believe, it can achieve.
-- Napoleon Hill

Discovering your inner strengths will provide new pathways toward reaching the goals which excite YOU. Finding your passion can circumvent feelings like Anhedonia and imposter syndrome. It will enable you to walk more boldly in your purpose.

You will begin to use:

1. **Self-reflection.** A reminder of strengths and resources used in the past to accomplish goals. The encouragement to know you can strategize a solution.
2. **Self-examination.** Inventory check of updated skills and resources that you can use to move forward. This will highlight underutilized strengths, support self-confidence, and uplift self-motivation to help reengage in a task expecting a better outcome.
3. **Self-efficacy.** The empowerment to move forward enables success and setbacks to occur without complete derailment of your goal. It reminds you that there is a next step you are equipped to try. If it is less than what you expected, you have the ability to go back and try another pathway. Or you can pause and start again later. If the outcome is better than expected, you can surpass self- obsession and keep moving

forward.

4. **Self-Advocacy.** Sustainability in your forward direction. Understanding and voicing your desires to yourself will help remind you of their consequential role in goal fulfillment. Sometimes we whisper or gloss over the value of a need thinking others will not comprehend its depth or importance. This is because we have not fully embraced the possibility of living the dream. Say it, write it, draw it, make a collage, or anything else that will help you see it coming to fruition. As you paint the picture for others, you will also advocate for the resources you need to fill any gaps in your plan. Others will align with you if they understand your request and have the bandwidth to assist.

Whose Expectations?

There will always be societal expectations. Some comparisons to others may be extended as teachable moments or motivation, not a burdensome weight. You may hear comments such as, "Your brother never did that." It happens in public settings, "I would never…" or "I have never seen someone…." These statements can exasperate insecurity and hinder a dream. Some people make cutting remarks, but the words of the wise bring healing. Proverbs 12:18 NLT.

If it is a challenge for others to understand their expectations are overwhelming you, two things will need to take place.

1. Coping mechanism. Find a way to decompress from the stress. This can come in the form of counting, listening to music, writing out your thoughts, closing your eyes or daydreaming you are at your favorite place. It just needs to be readily accessible, so that you can decompress quickly. Do your best to not let the stress define you.
2. Find a way to communicate how the comparisons make you feel. You can use a metaphor, comparative story or say it directly.

Sometimes you will have to repeat the message multiple times and use multiple methods to help others understand you. This book will provide some additional ideas on communication styles.

Comparisons can be a distortion of discernment. They are a perception of what has happened in the past and how it can be replayed in the future. If the person providing the comparison has a different history and contextual reference than the one you have lived with, then it may be time to develop a communication strategy. If they do not have the same skills or resources, you can seek support to help them see the value of your masked gifts and underutilized talents. This is not to abandon the goal. It is a pause to help uncover your best fit and most successful pathway to achieving your goal.

> You may have to fight a battle more than once to win it. -- Margaret Thatcher

Deconstructing Thoughts

Simply take the limits off. There are life experiences that can leave an indelible mark. It could be a joke, an accomplishment, an embarrassing moment, or one of your favorite school lessons. These experiences and the details in your recall of the event are inclusive of environmental stimuli. This can range from a hot beaming sun outside to a crying baby or a phone call that keeps dropping.

Growing up, I watched a futuristic show called The Jetsons. George Jetson drove a flying car. When we talked about the show at school, we would laugh about the silly concept of a flying car.

Repetitive talk and uniform socialization place boundaries on creativity and growth.

Luckily, the engineers at Klein Vision were able to deconstruct those limiting thoughts. They have built the Klein gyroplane. It is a car that flies on an unpowered motor. It uses the wind to lift the car off the ground.

As you uncover more about your character strengths in this book, you will have an opportunity to deconstruct limiting thoughts about yourself and continue to celebrate your awesomeness.

Cognitive Flexibility

This character strength highlights a person's nimbleness in unexpected situations. How quickly can you readjust to be productive in a surprising situation?

1. Practice Positive Thoughts. - Every new situation is an opportunity to grow and maybe help others around you grow and say thank you whenever possible.
2. Maintain an active network. Stay in touch with friends. Understand each-others interests and how you can help one another.
3. Chose to take a pause. This can vary from closing your eyes and thinking happy thoughts to excusing yourself for a walk and some fresh air. You understand the depth of what you will need to move forward.
4. Establish your norm for peace. Then create a compass and a roadmap to ensure you stay near or above your baseline/ starting point for continued clarity and joy.

It's in YOU. You have got this.

Chapter Two:
Communication Strengthening

Elevating Communication Confidence

Personal growth and evolution, the obtaining of new insight which affirms, alters, or deletes an existing belief, is ongoing. Whether you grow forward or sideways you are always growing. You may lose possessions and people, but you do not lose the experience and historical insight unless you have experienced a traumatic event which reduces memory or relies on implicit memory. You cannot remain stagnant because the world around you is continuously changing and your distinction of sight, sound, smell and touch are expanding. As you meet new people and date new persons, there will be new expectations, influences, norms, activities, interdependence, and requests.

The combination of your past experiences, current resources, and future expectations of fulfillment will influence the depth of your pursuit for consistency, collaboration, control, and change in future activities. As you infuse new knowledge into your current norms, stay in touch with your authentic self. Depth of self-understanding reduces communication apprehensiveness while enhancing passion, purpose, conviction, and clarity in spontaneous speech.

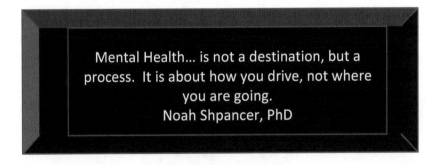

Mental Health... is not a destination, but a process. It is about how you drive, not where you are going.
Noah Shpancer, PhD

Take a deeper look within yourself

1. **Self- Awareness.** Valuing your unique gifts, strengths, and interests will help you to have greater control in customizing your best suited pathways to fulfillment and peace.
   *** **Self**-awareness includes taking a mental note of feeling overstressed after top life event stressors such as
   - Death or loss of a loved one
   - Divorce or Separation
   - Moving
   - Long-term Illness
   - Job loss

   A normal response to stress can be misinterpreted without an understanding of its context.

2. **Self- Help.** Expanding your use of your unique gifts, talents and resources to elevate your resilience and current situation.
3. **Self- Care.** Creating space to discover what replenishes your joy and actively doing it.
4. **Self- Starter.** Having the ambition, initiative, and tenacity to begin a new venture.

Taking an introspective inventory of your skills, interests, context, and priorities then effectively communicating them to collaborators can help reduce misinterpretations, time- delays, redundancy and more.

Sometimes collaborators, onlookers, and even clinicians may have a fixed mindset whereas your experience and insight have led you to a challenge mindset. Cultural, regional, economic, family dynamics and more can influence the agility of an onlooker's perceptions. Keep in mind there are 525,600 minutes in a year, still according to Cognitive Psychiatry of Chapel Hill, a psychiatrist can make a diagnosis and treatment plan within a 60-minute session.

An urgency to convey your vision to others before effectively communicating your pathway to your vision, and effectively having the listener agree that your plan is feasible, can be subjectively perceived an intrusion, perseveration, and nonadherence to the social rules for conversations – the **Diagnostic and Statistical Manual of Mental Disorders (DSM) 5** Pragmatic Language Disorder.

A DSM 5 Language Pragmatic Disorder diagnosis includes the clinician's valuation of social rule conduct

- An ability to change your language according to your audience
- Turn taking
- Body language
- Respecting personal space
- Knowing what to say, how to say it, and when to say it

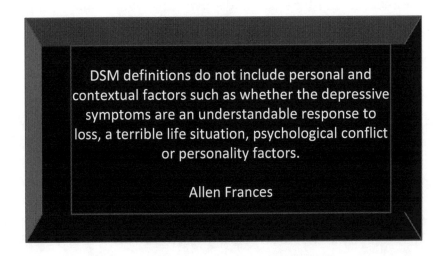

DSM definitions do not include personal and contextual factors such as whether the depressive symptoms are an understandable response to loss, a terrible life situation, psychological conflict or personality factors.

Allen Frances

Chapter Three:
Mindset

Personal prioritization of and accessibility to the components of complete wellness can guide mindset. Wellness characteristics include:
1. Emotional
2. Physical
3. Occupational
4. Social
5. Spiritual
6. Intellectual
7. Environmental
8. Financial

There are multiple types of mindsets. Three types which are frequently referenced are Fixed Mindset, Quantity Mindset and Challenge Mindset.

1. **Fixed Mindset** – this typically occurs when there is a dominant culture with homogeneous goals.

At least twice a year, my parents and I would travel to Pennsylvania Dutch Country for buggy rides, farm tours, groceries, and dinner. It is a beautiful Amish community where the locals drive horse driven carriages, wear full length attire and often farm for a living. In fact, they do not use modern day equipment for farming, and they have almost a 10 times lower obesity rate that the US population. Today's Anabaptist – related Pennsylvania Dutch Community culture and practices date back to the 16th century.

Many years ago, I visited Negril, Jamaica with several of my classmates. While in Negril, we talked to one of the local hair braiders every day. She told us about the great fresh seafood at her mother's restaurant. After eating at Rick's Café several nights, we figured we would go to her mother's restaurant that night.

When we arrived, we immediately noticed we were the only guests in the restaurant. So, we planned on getting out in an hour and making the beach party. In reality, the local culture was more relaxed, and time was not of the essence. They did not rush their food. Our dinner was not served until two hours after we sat down to eat. Once we were able to embrace the beauty of the local's peaceful pace, we were able to unwind and enjoy the amazing, distinct seasonings in our meal.

2. **Quantity Mindset** – this is when value is placed on accumulative historical experiences and historical data.

April Burrell is a former high school valedictorian and straight-A student at The University of Maryland Eastern Shore. She experienced an overwhelming trauma that eventually led her to being admitted to the psychiatric ward. Over almost twenty years of working with psychiatrists her condition grew to severe schizophrenia and she was unable to bath herself or communicate.

One of April's original physician's protégé met with April and reviewed her files. The physician then recruited 70 medical professionals from around the world, primarily neurologist and immunologists to uncover objective findings. A vast quantity of experts from across the world. They uncovered April Burrell had treatable Lupus. The same condition as Selina Gomez, Toni Braxton and Nick Cannon. After receiving treatments for Lupus, April Burrell is in rehabilitation center preparing for a life of greater independence.

Time constraints and reduced resources can force a quantity mindset. Imagine you are working for a hotel. The hotel has faced a 40% drop in overnight guests due to the loud construction noise outside. At the same time, you have had to extend refunds and lower prices due to due to customer complaints. If any of the available hotel rooms are not filled on a particular night, example October 20th, then you can never obtain the revenue for that room night again. Therefore, the front desk is in a quantity mindset each night the hotel is not at 100% occupancy. A hotel's attempt to sell 100% of their rooms every night, is why you will find last minute deals on hotel stays.

3. **Challenge Mindset** – this is when fortitude and agility allow a person to view challenges as an opportunity to create new pathways and redesign existing pathways to success. Going beyond status quo and complacency to innovation and sustainable solutions.

Emotional Challenge Mindset

Dr. Nadine Burke Harris received many requests to diagnose Oakland, California students with ADHD. The US has a 1 in 9 ratio of persons diagnosed with ADHD whereas the world has a 1 in 20 rate of ADHD. A lot of kids were being referred to her for ADHD but after a thorough diagnosis she realized she could not diagnose them with ADHD. Instead, she treated most of her referrals without extending an ADHD diagnosis.

She went beyond status quo and was appointed the Surgeon General for California.

Emotional Challenge Mindset

Dr. Patricia Resick developed Cognitive Processing Therapy (CPT) in the 1980's to treat persons who had experienced rape and other interpersonal trauma. Clients transition from overwhelming perceptions of guilt and blame to factual understandings and balance.

In a Duke University clinical study of Dr. Resick's approach to addressing PTSD, within 6 weeks 40% of group therapy participants and one-half of one-to-one patients no longer met the diagnostic criteria for PTSD.

Environmental Challenge Mindset

Michael Phelps kindergarten teacher said Micheal will "never be able to focus on anything." He was an active child who had difficulty sitting and loved to stir mischief. Two years later, his parents divorced and he began taking swim lessons with his sisters. He hated it. He started off with the backstroke because he did not like getting his face wet. Once he mastered the back stroke, he loved swimming and there was no turning back. While swimming, the tensions of the world - persistent bullying, parents' divorce, having a different energy than peers and negative feedback from teachers – would dissipate as he swam for hours. Michael was in control.

In the sixth grade, Michael was diagnosed with ADHD. Michael and his mother were determined to challenge the perceived limitations of his diagnosis. A team of individuals worked with Michael to help him excel. Michael competed in the Olympics at age 15.

Michael Phelps continues to challenge the perceived limitations of people who learn differently. He understands how an environment's physical and emotional clutter can impact a person's ability to find balance and control. He felt a peace and control in the water that would better enable him to obtain, retain and apply new information. The Michael Phelps Foundation partners with the Special Olympics to train coaches on how to coach persons, like Michael, who have special needs.

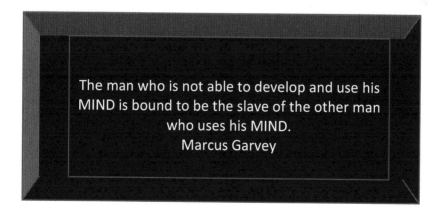

Occupational Challenge Mindset

David Steward was a top salesman at Federal Express. His excellence in sales led to him to receive the Salesman of the Year award. The award included a listing in the Federal Express Hall of Fame and an engraved silver ice bucket. When he looked inside the empty ice bucket, he saw emptiness and confinement. The vision gave Stewart a challenge mindset. He challenged the concept of working extremely hard, achieving excellence, and ending with a feeling of confinement and emptiness.

After the awards ceremony, Steward borrowed $2,000 from his father to start a company. Today, Steward is the chairman and founder of World Wide Technology. He is worth over $7.6 billion dollars.

Intellectual Challenge Mindset

Dr. Susan Swedo of the National Institute of Mental Health and Autism sought to reduce the chances of human error in diagnosing OCD, ADHD, and Autism by looking at objective and tangible data which provided greater translatable insight. Her desire to cure not just mange these conditions has led to patient's loss of diagnostic symptoms, full treatment coverage mandates in select states, and transitions from a life of dependency to college graduation.

The United States has a 1 in 36 rate of autism vs the world's average rate of 1 in 100 and other wealthy countries average of 1 in 138.

Physical Challenge Mindset

Tom Stoltman. Stoltman, Winner of the World's Strongest Man hated going to the gym. At the age of five he was diagnosed with autism. Teachers told him he was not going to do anything with his life and he was continuously bullied by other students. His mother recorded videos of

Tom's work at home. His teachers were receptive to the videos and became agile in their teaching styles.

Stoltman used his tunnel vision focus to repeatedly surpass his weight bearing expectations. His goal is to become an ambassador for autism.

Chapter Four:
Self-Assessment

Self-assessments can become the dais for sustainable self-affirmation. Positive outlooks impact the way we process change, perceive limitations, embrace character strengths, and more. After high school, cognitive tests are extended to athletes and persons who are building careers in corporate America to ascertain their approach to problem-solving.

Some of the frequently referenced self-assessment tests include the optional Wonderlic Contemporary Cognitive Ability Test and the S2 Cognition Test for NFL Combine invitees, the Athletic Intelligence Quotient for the NBA plus several other professional sports leagues, the Enneagram Personality Test, and 89 of the Fortune 100 companies use the Myers Briggs Type Indicator (MBTI).

The MBTI is a self-assessment, a personal preference test, which implies the values a person will use in their decision-making decision process. When their preferences are understood, appreciated, and put into action there is an internal reward. This type of satisfaction supports increased re-engagement, commitment, purpose, and self-worth.

These tests can provide a baseline, but context is essential.

One of the significant challenges with viewing these scores in isolation is the ever-changing context. In grad school, I learned that no two teaching environments are ever the same. The slightest variance can make a difference.

A recent or still managing life-altering situation, such as death, marriage, blended families, relocation, divorce, co- parenting, car accident, and more, can skew these types of life and opportunity-determining test scores. Even the more subtle "should" and "ought to" from loved ones can create hesitancy or distort a more accurate response. These instances can challenge readiness through emotional regulation blurring current sentiments with continued and more authentic perceptions in test responses.

Did you know not fully recovering from the flu, chickenpox, and other illnesses can impact your readiness? One example is PANDAS/PANS.

Rheumatologist

Immunologist

Hematologist

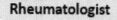

Neurologist

Sometimes people will reach an impasse and need additional assistance with readiness. Tracking your progress towards a goal can help you understand even subtle changes in skill strengths and interests.

One example of a medical condition that impacts readiness and can be misdiagnosed is PANDAS/ PANS. It is a condition where infections cause a person's immune system to direct its pruning on the brain instead of the disease. This leads to impairments in problem solving, speech, and overall engagement. Noted social behavior challenges include sudden anger, compulsion, eating restrictions, obsession, rage, screaming, and violence.

Pediatrician

Oncologist

Psychiatrist

Psychologist

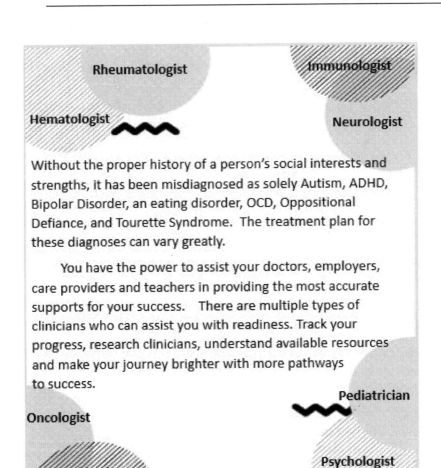

Without the proper history of a person's social interests and strengths, it has been misdiagnosed as solely Autism, ADHD, Bipolar Disorder, an eating disorder, OCD, Oppositional Defiance, and Tourette Syndrome. The treatment plan for these diagnoses can vary greatly.

You have the power to assist your doctors, employers, care providers and teachers in providing the most accurate supports for your success. There are multiple types of clinicians who can assist you with readiness. Track your progress, research clinicians, understand available resources and make your journey brighter with more pathways to success.

Taking time to create a baseline of test scores, character strengths, communication skills, and interests then periodically checking your test scores will provide you pathways to move beyond dysergy, the "idea that the whole is lesser than the sum of its parts," to a better understanding of how the things around you are impacting your joy. It will assist you with insight into mandatory test score results as well as answering the 5 W's In your decision- making process.

Are you ready? Let's go. Let's go!

> If you don't understand yourself, you don't understand anybody else. -- Nikki Giovanni

Self–Assessment of Transparency and Strengths-Based Goal Analysis

Today's Date

Balance can be obscure for taskmasters. They are dependable, disciplined, and skilled, and everyone expects the best of them.

Onlookers are people who are only capturing a snapshot of your day or 60 minutes of a 24-hour day. They cannot see inside another person's mind. They cannot see the multiple layers of sacrifice and commitment you experience in delivering excellence. If a person does not understand what's important to them, they can get into a rut of solely taking on other tasks.

What if someone else's list of tasks and your needs differ? What if your busyness prevents you from uncovering and addressing your needs, while everyone around you excels? One way to circumvent this cycle is by developing a baseline self- assessment to gain a comprehensive insight into what's important to you.

This is an ongoing self-assessment. You can start now or once you have read half of this book. It's a point of reference that can be used to check the progress you are making toward your goal.

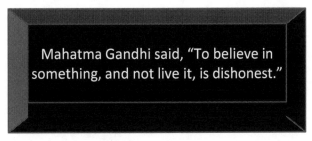

Mahatma Gandhi said, "To believe in something, and not live it, is dishonest."

Celebrate the obstacles you have overcome.

Celebrate your wisdom and awareness of the pathways you do not want to revisit.

Celebrate your advancements forward.

Influence and Impact – Influence and Impact – Write an elevator pitch about yourself in a few sentences. Your pitch should include four items:
1. Info about you - name, location, school, or job
2. Skills
3. Goal
4. How you will feel when you accomplish your goal

In my experience with coaching and teaching, students and clients have felt unmotivated to try based on obstacles. They could list things that were hindering them and how those things made them feel in great detail. After they exhausted their list, I would get them to start listing the things they enjoyed. The list of things they enjoyed was far away or just not something they could access today.

Since the things they enjoyed were not available today, we started working on timetables, milestones, and pathways for them to reach their goals. Well, once they saw their dream was attainable, their interest and effort in daily activities changed. They were ready.

Obtainable goals that match your skills and interest always supersede obstacles. Just ask the NBA basketball player Michael Jordan who was cut from his high school basketball team.

Take time to understand your skills, interests, and resources. Then map out a plan to achieve your dreams in a way that is fun for you.

Give yourself permission to do great things and have fun.

Consider what you write in a draft; you can write in pen and use cross-outs, or note that it is a draft at the top of your screen before you begin typing. Include your vision of how you will impact or influence others' lives. As you begin to uncover new collaborations, resources, skills, and more you may have to edit your pitch.

_____

_____
_____
_____
_____
_____
_____
_____
_____
_____

The number seven traditionally is a sign of fullness. The self-assessment questions below provide an opportunity for you to build your pathway to fullness.

List up to seven ways your vision will improve your own life.

_____	_____
_____	_____
_____	_____
_____	_____
_____	_____
_____	_____
_____	_____

Now that you have made your list of (up to) seven, circle the top three items in your list that benefit you. Then circle the top three that will benefit others.

List up to seven collaborations you will form to make your vision a reality.

_____
_____
_____
_____
_____
_____
_____

List up to seven skills you have or will learn to GROW your ability to make your vision a reality.

_____	_____
_____	_____
_____	_____
_____	_____
_____	_____
_____	_____
_____	_____

List up to seven resources you use or expand to make your vision a reality.

_____	_____
_____	_____
_____	_____
_____	_____
_____	_____
_____	_____
_____	_____

Place the letter N next to items with a current need, but you will have to allocate time to explain the urgency or skill you need to acquire.

Optimal Ending. What is an optimal ending for you for this phase of personal or business development? When will you end, pivot, or celebrate?

Divide your goal into seven phases.

Describe Phase One.
_____
_____
_____
_____
_____
_____
_____
_____

Describe Phase Two.
_____
_____
_____
_____
_____
_____
_____
_____

Describe Phase Three.
_____
_____
_____
_____
_____
_____
_____
_____

Describe Phase Four.

Describe Phase Five.

Describe Phase Six.

Describe Phase Seven.

Additional Notes

Likert Type Scale. What seven ongoing questions will you ask your collaborators and yourself to check progress, engagement, and effectiveness?

Create an ongoing list of resources (persons, places, or supplies) you will need to accomplish your goal. Place an asterisk beside the items that require external collaborations or consultants.

PERSON (S)	PLACE	SUPPLIES
_____	_____	_____
_____	_____	_____
_____	_____	_____
_____	_____	_____
_____	_____	_____
_____	_____	_____

Discovery. Dedicate time for daily discovery and self-reflection.

Reporting / Recoding strategy

_____
_____
_____
_____
_____
_____
_____
_____

Affirming, Adjusting, and Advancing Agility Process

_____
_____
_____
_____
_____
_____
_____
_____
_____
_____
_____
_____
_____
_____
_____
_____
_____

Chapter Five:
Edge- Unmask Your Greatness

While I was growing up, my mom taught me to find the good in everyone. If a playmate seemed sad, I had to stop playing, ask them how they were feeling, and listen to them. I became a master at finding greatness in others, but I did not have a clue about how to find it in me. Talk about burnout. I did not know how to ask for or where to seek the affirmation that would encourage me during tough times.

The 2023 Heath Day- Harris Poll reported 63% of doctors stated they are feeling burnout at work. If they have been professionally trained to hear and manage the concerns of their patient and feel worn down, then it is possible for others without similar professional schooling and training to get burned out. Pace yourself. Dr. Vytas Vaitkus studied physicians at SUNY Downstate and discovered the importance of downtime for physicians.

He incorporated more fun activities for the team of doctors and noticed how smiling helps to dissipate feelings of burnout. Challenges fall upon everyone, and people are pulled in many directions daily. Self-assessments will help you, a nonprofessional, understand when you need to press "pause" on all the external demands and ask, "What do I need to laugh right now?"

A recent study showed 1 in 10 physicians have suicidal ideations. The average doctor sees 20 patients a day; therefore, in a 51-hour work week, a doctor may see more than 100 patients a week. During their usually short appointments, doctors must figure out a lot of patient history.

Imagine the fatigue of patients not telling them everything or the doctor not understanding what they are saying, and their symptoms get worse. Many people, even close relatives, and friends can misinterpret what you are saying because their years and layers of experience can be completely different from yours.

As referenced in the burnout statistics, many doctors are hurt when they are unable to help their patients heal as planned. They spend many years in school and lots of dollars on education with the goal of helping their patients heal. Every patient's success is their success. Understand and keep a record of changes in your health. Reporting these items can help relay the detailed sequence of events that brought you to their office. Clearer communication can help to increase appointment efficiency and improve treatment plan accuracy and overall health outcomes.

It's time to go beyond imagining success and use your character strengths to *make* success happen.
Let's make it stick.

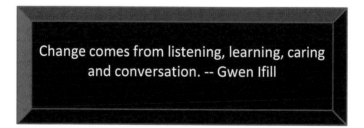

Change comes from listening, learning, caring and conversation. -- Gwen Ifill

One day my director gave me the Myers Briggs Assessment.

My score was an ENTP. The E was extremely low. She kept saying I was a classic ENTP, provided opportunities to highlight an ENTP's skill set, and cheered me on as I nailed each task.

It was the **first** time I knew my director understood me, and I began to understand myself. I did not have to call her for affirmation because every task she gave me was another opportunity for success.

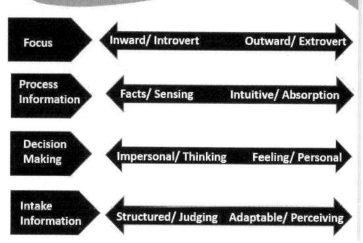

The Myers Briggs Personality Combination Types

- INTJ - The Strategist
- INTP - The Engineer
- ENTJ - The Chief
- ENTP - The Originator
- INFJ - The Confidant
- INFP - The Dreamer
- ENFJ - The Mentor
- ENFP - The Advocate
- ISTJ – The Examiner
- ISFJ – The Defender
- ESTJ - The Overseer
- ESFJ - The Supporter
- ISTP - The Craftsman
- ISFP - The Artist
- ESTP - The Persuader
- ESFP - The Entertainer

A work and school environment which compliments your personality type can

1. Remind you of your excellence
2. Provide opportunities that highlight your skills
3. Assist with obtaining, retaining, and applying new information
4. Help you understand your pace or workflow
5. Support your intrinsic values
6. Increase your engagement and fulfillment
7. Enhance your overall quality of life

Conversely, if it is the opposite of your personality type, it can drain you. Taking the time to discover your interests will help you to communicate your needs more effectively, be heard, and uncover multiple constructive pathways to move FORWARD. These benefits are amplified when you can communicate your values effectively and understand another person.

Understanding the interests of yourself and others can circumvent frequent periods of burnout. Acknowledging others may have different perceptions, expectations, and work habits than you, will allow you to see how their unique gifts assist your environment. You will be able to encourage them and yourself as you authentically walk bolder in self-efficacy.

Communication is more than the words we say each day. Words are a low conveyor of message meaning. They are only 7% of communication. Someone can say "Thank you" with the worst attitude and roll their eyes. Sometimes people will give a response based on another person's expectations. It may not be because they are happy to respond. Paying attention to more than one form of communication can help a person possess greater insight into how they should respond next.

Dr. Albert Mehrabian, a psychology professor, created the 7-38-55 Rule. It explains how communication is expressed and received in more than one format. He emphasizes looking at three communication indicators - body language, tone, and words. This approach provides a clearer picture of the intended message and desired response. Masked sentiments can be hidden if an audience solely focuses on words.

Acknowledging 55% of communication emotions expressed through a person's body movements can assist with understanding the whole picture. Have you ever listened to the TV or something on the computer? After hearing something of interest, you stopped what you were doing to look at the screen. Seeing what you heard took your level of understanding to a new level. Or someone providing a detailed description of a big smile, bold stance, puzzled face, or arching back move in a new dance. What you see can change what you perceive.

Example. If you ask someone, "How are you?" Then they respond, "I am great." It will also help to observe their body language during the response. If their posture does not match the confidence of "Great," then it could be time to pause, ask about other tasks, and learn what is preoccupying their thoughts.

While conversing, listen for tone of voice. It is 38% of communication. Would you believe your words are only 7% of communication emotions?

In the book *Men Are from Mars, Women Are from Venus*, author John Gray mentions, "Women are like waves.... demanding to be heard from time to time." Incorporating all three forms of communication could help to ensure that she is being heard. This example highlights the visual benefits of face-to-face communication.

Seeing a person's face and body language helps to define their message. Phone communication allows you to hear the tone of the speaker and provide a more complete picture of their intentions.

A Highly Sensitive Person (HSP) has the gifted ability to use multiple communication forms simultaneously. They are able to grasp a deeper and more empathetic meaning of another

person's comments through the use of their five senses. This means they may be able to hear distant sounds more clearly than the people near them. This can be a great thing or a challenge. Imagine the ability to hear the conversation next to you, airplanes flying nearby, the fan on a generator, the school crossing guard's whistle, and car brakes at the same time and at the same volume. If they are unable to effectively explain this to listeners, striving to live up to the expectations of others could be a challenge. Having keen visual skills with the ability to read lips could be difficult if the environment is not affirming.

One thing people with HSP may have to manage is an itchy aversion to clothing. Some fabrics feel scratchy and overwhelmingly irritable. The Superhero Superman had the strength to overcome many challenges yet Kryptonite debilitated him. It left him weak while he fought to get away from it. This irritable distraction from Kryptonite describes the pain someone with HSP can experience the moment they walk outside, take off their headphones, take off their sunglasses, or wear a nametag. An unawareness or mislabeling of these symptoms can delay a person from walking in their true self. HSP enables greatness in its best- suited environment.

> Poets can tell the truth as they see it. It's the author's story, the author's voice. -- Nikki Giovanni

Chapter Six:
Sidelined- I Never Had the Whole Picture

Partially accurate assessments can have limited, unfulfilling, and harmful long-term effects. We often hear, "No question is a bad question,"," but what if the person you are asking does not know the answer? Or, what if they are so entrenched and comfortable with tradition that their solutions are ineffective? What if the person asking and answering the question is you?

It's Time to Fill in the Gap

OK, let us transition to a deeper understanding of what is important to you.

Sometimes, when a person tells someone else about their challenges, people will tell them, "Fake it until you make it." If you conduct a self-assessment and you believe what you are facing is temporary, then this method can work. It is essentially a band-aid for short-term, or interval challenges. These events are small interruptions or delays as you strive to reach a goal.

After being sidetracked, finding the sustainable motivation to reengage can be a journey. A transition leap can be a purposeful tool used to get you started. A transition is an intentional turn and can be a 180-degree shift from the direction you are currently going. This type of leap requires self-efficacy as you force yourself out of the comfort of old routines to align with something new and more promising.

The key to a leap is direction, force, and a balanced landing. If one of these three components is missing, instead of moving forward a person could move in full circles. A 360-degree turn, more than once, can surface the recycling of unsuccessful habits and disengagement. Going beyond faking it to clearly understand and communicate your needs, can help your crowd of peers best understand how they can partner with you and support you. You will be walking in your authentic strengths.

Since 1994, I have coached a diverse group of people. Two sentiments have been consistent. A strengths-based approach leads to greater self-confidence, engagement, and overall success. Having a defined purpose or goal helps to surpass any obstacles.

Many standardized tests can provide insight into a person's communication, and social engagement styles in order, and help to establish fulfilling goals. Some results may be distorted based on environmental stimuli or the test provider. If a student or employee relocates to a new area, adjusting to a new environment can be challenging. In my YouTube interview with former Professional Basketball Player Samarie Walker, she highlighted how her homesickness during college caused anxiety and led to her quick transfer to colleges.

According to the National Institute of Health, 94% of college students experience homesickness during their first 10 weeks of college. The unfamiliarity can lead to a shock that impacts academic performance.

If the test results are interpreted without understanding the events and items which may have altered your typical response, they can lead a person on a narrow path with setbacks and brick walls. Some situations are temporary. The anticipation of getting out of that temporary situation can impact a person's focus and authentic response. Self-awareness will let you know how your focus is being impacted. It will give you the opportunity to more clearly explain how far out of your normal range you are feeling and ask for assistance when needed.

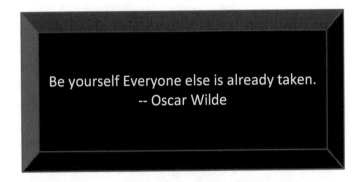

> Be yourself Everyone else is already taken.
> -- Oscar Wilde

Conversely, a familiar testing environment and the familiarity of a proctor can favorably impact test scores. Thomas Alva Edison's school sent a letter to his mother stating Thomas was mentally deficient and could not attend school anymore. His mother viewed him as having a different learning style from his peers rather than embracing the incorrect assumption that he was incapable of learning.

Thomas Alva Edison's accomplishments changed the narrative of his life. Today, many consider him one of the most brilliant people of the 20th century, proceeding to obtain 1,093 US patents.

Nine-time Grammy Award Winning Producer, Marcus Boyd, did not begin speaking in full sentences until after age 20. "It's never too late to understand and strengthen a mind. Whether or not they have learning problems, students need to know how their minds work—learn about learning while they are learning," said Dr. Mel Levine at the University of North Carolina at Chapel Hill.

A move forward will also require a look inward.

Before expanding your audience and inviting others to join you during your journey, it is essential to understand how you perceive yourself vs. what others may perceive you are saying. This is not to delay the process- it is to make sure the steps of progression and final results reflect your authentic self.

Establishing your goals and time availability will create more work-life balance as you form new partnerships. This will help to manage everyone's expectations and circumvent burnout. You, your purpose, and your pathway to success are distinct.

It should be customized because there is only one you. Your contributions are unique.

Some audiences are not going to be prepared for your insight. That's okay. When you find the right environment and form the right partnerships, you will have the ability to open the hearts and minds of others to develop more effective solutions.

Once you begin to move forward, you will face new challenges and resistance. Having a solid foundation will help you to stay resilient and focused. It will provide self-affirmation reminding you of your nimbleness and the resources available to achieve success.

If you experience challenges moving forward, you will not be alone. Take the time needed to find your best solution. Traditionally, college students would graduate in four years. Today, they are spending more time defining themselves and their career goals before they graduate.

A 2022 National Science Clearinghouse Research Center reports 62.3 percent of undergraduate students in the U.S. completed their degree programs within six years of enrolling in college.

More than 75% of Division One and 50% of Division Two college basketball players believe they have a chance to play professional basketball. The competition, injuries, and plays may impact an athlete's ability to play in season games. The reality for college athletes is 1.2% will play for a National Basketball Association (NBA) team.

Playing for a professional team is not impossible- it requires discipline and an understanding of your strengths. Making your basketball shots count when you get the ball and advancing the football toward your opponent's end goal requires playing to your strengths. Terry Porter, the Division Three University of Wisconsin at Stevens Point basketball point guard, understood his strengths. He played for 17 years in the NBA.

Challenges are inevitable. Mastering your strengths will help you view obstacles as pathways to a greater opportunity and a time to exercise your strengths.

If you have a personal goal, then you owe it to yourself to investigate the pathways that match your strengths to achieve it. You can move forward by activating and celebrating your gifts and uniqueness.

Anthony "Spud" Webb, who, at five feet, seven inches was one of the shortest men to play in the NBA, was granted the opportunity to play on his high school basketball team, after two of his starting teammates did not complete the required physical exam. Those two teammates created a pathway for Webb to highlight his skills.

Spud prepared himself for the opportunity and performed solidly as an individual and team player to land a starting position on his team. He just kept looking forward. Webb defied a naysayer sports analyst by leading the NBA in free-throw shooting and winning a slam dunk contest. His gift was more than physical agility. He had exemplary problem-solving skills and was determined to succeed.

Pursuing a vision that is important to you, can stir a new sense of passion and purpose. The excitement of continuously surpassing obstacles that onlookers may have considered immovable is euphoric. The vision of your end goal becomes brighter and more defined because you are setting the course. You can customize incorporating what you need to succeed. This boost can also help you mentor others with similar goals along the way. First, transition towards your goal. Then build yourself up and allow affirming persons to help you. After you find your way or develop a roadmap remember to help build others up.

> The idea that men are created free and equal is both true and misleading: men are created different; they lose their social freedom and their individual autonomy in seeking to become like each other. David Reisman, *The Lonely Crowd*

Task Analysis

Strategic planning helps enhance collaborations, support, influence, and target audience engagement, to further the longevity/ sustainability of an accomplished goal. It includes your skills, resources, and environment. Its enemy is familiarity and boredom.

One way to increase excitement about an activity is to use task analysis. Without it, we might miss opportunities for innovation and celebration. Think of all the additions to the iPhone. Apple reviewed the process required to complete a goal and found a way to improve the outcome. They examined each step. After they improved a step in the process, they created a new iPhone product.

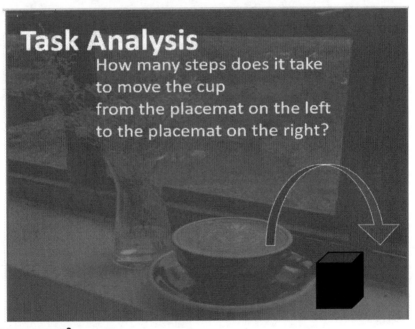

What is your answer?

Typically, when I ask people this question, their response is either statement one or statement two in the list below. The correct answer in Task Analysis is eight.

1. Look at the cup. If you are looking at the cup you can avoid <u>reaching</u> in the wrong direction, knocking over the flower vase, spilling water on the table, and staining the wood.
2. Reach for the cup. If you reach for it, then you <u>grab</u> it and complete the task. Looking at it may not move it.
3. Grab the cup. If you do not grab the cup, it may fall out of your hands when you try to <u>lift</u> it. Or it may be more prone to spill.
4. Lift the cup with your hand (s). The cup needs to go over the black cube to move <u>right</u> and avoid clashing and possibly spilling.
5. Move your arm right, with the cup in your hand. This will help you <u>place</u> the cup in its designated position.
6. Place the cup in the new location on the table. The cup should be resting on the table before you <u>let go</u> to avoid a spill.
7. Let go of the cup. This will enable you to get <u>ready</u> for whatever comes next.
8. Place your arm and hand back in the ready position.

This may seem tedious, but the steps in a strategic plan are interdependent. You may pause or rest in between steps to make sure you have everything you need for the next step. You may even repeat a step to make sure you have the best platform to advance. The key to effectiveness, efficiency, vibrancy, and fulfillment is completing each step.

You deserve the excitement of an accomplished, vibrant, awe-struck dream. Don't settle. If needed, adjust your strategic plan so that you can move forward confidently.

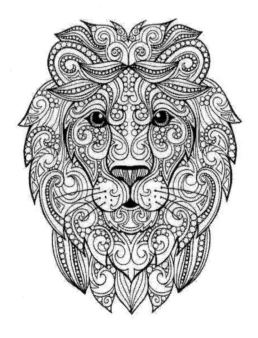

Illustrations by Eric Ottinger and iStock by Getty Images

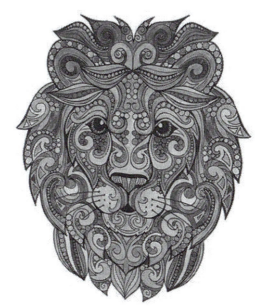

Utilizing the 5Ws (who, what, when, where, and why) and how personal filters will elevate you to a greater self- efficacy

Journalists are tasked with answering the 5Ws in every story they report.

- Who - describe the character of the persons in the story.
- What - describe what happened or is going to happen.
- When - describe the timeline of events
- Where - describe the location of the story.
- Why - describe the big picture of the story.

If a reporter were to interview you today, are you ready to answer the 5Ws about you? How will you define yourself?

This chapter provides exercises that will help you customize your responses to the 5Ws. This response can also be used as you seek a mentor and form new partnerships. Utilizing the 5Ws (who, what, when, where, and why) and how personal filters will elevate you to greater self-efficacy.

Chapter Seven:
Who I Enjoy

Your unique character gives you and your audience an advantage in every encounter.

Sometimes a person will temper this gift when trying to conform to their environment. Your character traits are like muscles. They are active when you are moving forward toward your goals. When these character muscles are inactive, they develop atrophy. This stiffness means you will have to spend more hours stretching a great deal, more than unusual, to get out of stagnation. Over-stretching can cause more harm than good so find your pace.

Utilizing your strengths in an affirming environment, your value is seen and acknowledged, you will invite more chances to influence and lead. One of the things many of my students and young adults have told me is they are running exhausted from trying to meet societal expectations. If a person is weighed down by lifting everyone else up 90% and you are lifted up 10% it can cause a person to experience feelings of anxiousness and boredom. They become tired of explaining and compromising because their energy is being depleted.

In an affirming environment, people encourage and highlight one another's strengths. You see them both getting stronger - it's not one-sided. One person who comes to mind when I think of unique personalities is Rahm Emanuel, who, when representing an Illinois congressional district, was as visible as his party's presidential candidate– Barack Obama. He was well-versed on all subject matters and had his candidate's support, so he spent a lot of time on camera making very pointed comments about issues. He was passionate, intentional, engaging, entertaining, and a risk-taker. There was never a dull moment when Emanuel spoke.

Former President Obama is even-keeled, humble, and kind. He possesses the cognitive flexibility to effectively manage interruptions. During his campaign, there were several times he had to shift gears and use his diplomatic skills to soften one of Emanuel's comments. The polarized contrast between the two personalities kept voters informed, excited, and engaged.

Some people, myself included, could not wait to turn on the news to hear Emmanuel's comment of the day. His brevity, high energy, and arrogance helped to get inconsistent and younger voters engaged in the campaign process. Obama's ease with storytelling and attentiveness helped to comfort senior and traditional voters who were alarmed by Emanuel's direct approach. The polarization of unique communication styles between Emanuel and Obama kept many audiences picking sides on their favorite and engaged in the political race.

Emmanuel's personality was too big to be boxed. Embracing his strengths and media attraction provided Obama more room to discern which topics to highlight and which pathways to proceed. It was a dynamic balance of character with diverse delivery styles that offered journalists robust content to report.

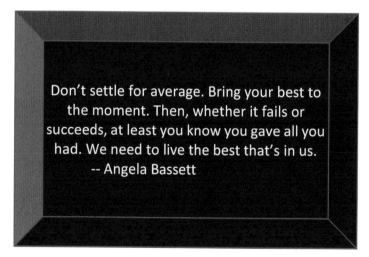

Don't settle for average. Bring your best to the moment. Then, whether it fails or succeeds, at least you know you gave all you had. We need to live the best that's in us.
  -- Angela Bassett

Sometimes your ability to influence others is too big for some, not all, audiences to comprehend.

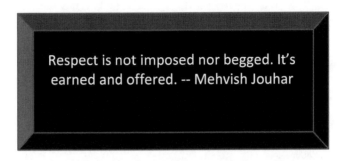

Positive Psychology's 24 Character Strengths

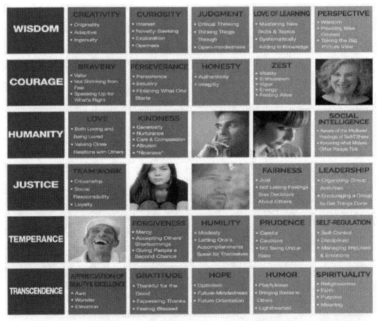

Utilizing your dominant character strengths can help maximize the endorphins you release when you finish a project.

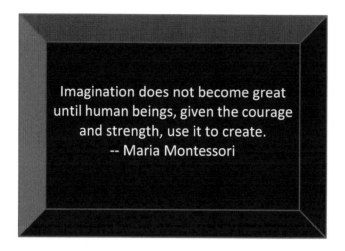

Projects with a high virtue value for you, offer more fulfillment and a greater desire to reengage. When possible, prioritize including activities with high intrinsic value in your schedule.

Chapter Eight:
What I Think

My workday in Midtown Manhattan typically started with coffee at the NY Hilton. After weeks of only hearing French spoken in the NY Hilton's Ladies' room, I asked Stephanie, one of my hotel colleagues, if she had experienced the same thing at the NY Hilton. She responded, "Kellye, they have a contract with FAM Tour operators in France. The hotel will have over 100 guests from France for many nights. You see them before they begin their sight-seeing tour of the city."

Wow! This was something new to me. So many people from France in one place. I immediately thought I am going to stop by the bathroom, every day, to see if I can learn something new about France. Maybe I can learn a few new words and practice using the words I learned in high school. I just kept thinking about opportunities and possibilities.

Growing up, my dad and I would read about international cities in the World Book Encyclopedia. Since I have not had the chance to travel overseas, I marvel over conversations about foreign countries. What excites you? The Enneagram Personality Assessment is a tool that can be used to find out more about what motivates you. This is the link to a free Enneagram Personality Test

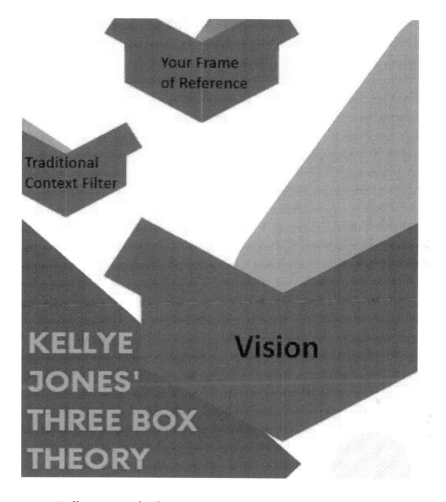

Kellye Jones' Three Box Theory. A vision is accomplished through a series of steps forward.

Life's lessons help us figure out what we would like to do in the future. At an impasse, we may contact those closest to us for help. Despite their unfamiliarity with the subject matter, they know how to comfort our fears, so we keep them on our emergency speed dial list. Mixing the feeling of comfort with a need for topical insight can stunt or even stop progress.

Your emergency contacts may see your vision as impossible based on their life experiences. They may think, since I have never seen it done before it's not necessary. Your moving forward may be the catalyst for your friends dreaming bigger dreams. So, keep your excitement and keep pressing forward. As you become more familiar with your unique character strengths, you will find more persons with similar values and broader experiences to help you uncover more pathways to success.

Our self-efficacy influences how we process events and move forward.

Stuck – Societal Expectations

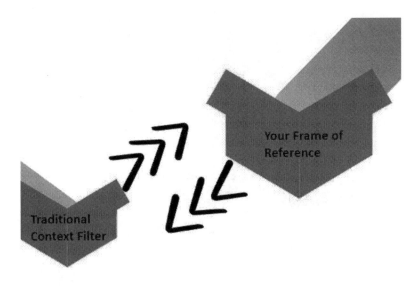

It is easier to generalize when people have busy schedules and historical insight. So, in seconds a situation or person's action can be misjudged.

A Microsoft Corp. study revealed the average human attention span is 8 seconds. This can lead to shortcuts and the habit of recycling outdated practices.

Confirmation bias is when you form a favorable or unfavorable opinion about something, and you use new information to affirm your existing opinion. Let's say something is red shoes. As you meet more people and have new experiences you receive new information about red shoes. Whether the new information says red shoes are great or red shoes are bad, you will only believe the information which confirms your original opinion about red shoes. The information which negates your original belief, you will find ways to discredit it because acceptance would require you to review all of your old beliefs. It's just easier and time-saving to stick with traditions.

According to a US Department of Health and Human Services Agency for Healthcare Research report, there are 7 - 12 million annual medical misdiagnoses.

The primary reason for these misdiagnoses is asymptomatic or unfamiliar symptoms. Time limitations and generalizations can leave a person, even a physician, using confirmation bias and generalizations to fill in gaps of missing patient information and best manage time constraints.

As mental health cases increase and more rare health conditions are uncovered, there are more variables to securing the most effective treatment plan. One way to assist your care provider is to ensure you are able to accurately answer standard doctor's office and Emergency Room questions.

Psychoneuroimmunology (PIN) or (PEN)

Psychoneuroimmunology highlights the interdependence of psychological reasoning and the cognitive development, the physical and visible components of the central nervous system, the objectively measurable components of the immune system. It includes responses to environmental stimuli (sensations that are not created by oneself) and the delayed-onset of a condition.

The **Diagnostic and Statistical Manual (DSM-5)** has a new broadened criteria for diagnosing mental health conditions. The redefining of criteria has enabled some practices to extend a mental health diagnosis within 60 minutes. The quick turnaround emphasizes the critical importance of staying ready to provide comprehensive self-reporting.

Self- Reports to physicians should include items such as context, prior success (social, physical and cognitive), as well as the onset, frequency, duration and intensity of new challenges. During the 525,600 minutes in a year 0r 262,800 minutes in six months, by forgetting or eliminating these events in your self-report you could negatively impact your diagnosis.

ADHD has been mistakenly diagnosed for persons with PTSD. The symptoms for both of the diagnosis include hyperactivity, inattention and impulsivity. An awareness of life events could increase the accuracy of a diagnosis and effectiveness of a treatment plan.

Vitamin C deficiency is also associated with a decreased level of attention.

Researchers from the Geha Mental Health Center, Mount Sinai, and Cambridge Health Alliance uncovered a higher rate of immunodeficiency amongst children with ADHD vs the general population of youth.

Autism has been mistakenly diagnosed for patients with Complex Post Traumatic Stress Disorder Syndrome. The symptoms for both include impaired communication skills, social awkwardness / social anxiety and pervasiveness.

Persons with PTSD continuously replay a situation to gain control over an external event. Dr. Allen Frances was one of the physicians who led the DSM-4 's broadening of the criteria for autism.

Today, he apologizes for lessening the criteria stating, he is "very sorry for the over-diagnosis of autism." A recent Rutgers University study noted the 500% increase in autism cases in the US.

The US has a rate of 1 in 36 persons diagnosed with autism. The world has a rate of 1 in 100 persons diagnosed with autism.

Mild brain injury and delayed- onset PTSD include symptoms of delayed or impaired speech, social awkwardness / challenges with social judgement and repetitiveness. Autism is present at birth. So, a traumatic event should not cause **adulthood autism** but it can mimic autism.

Bipolar has been mistakenly diagnosed as Complex PTSD in the absence of contextual information. Both of the diagnosis have symptoms which include positive and negative excitement.

Depression or Anxiety as a result of B12 deficiency. B12 helps the central nervous system with mood regulation. It enhances dopamine, the "feel good" hormone and serotonin for cognition and memory levels. Some foods which provide B12 include eggs, sardines, cheese, tuna and salmon.

Complex PTSD (CPTSD) is the repetitive or prolonged exposure to trauma. It causes a physical change, neurological change, to your brain's structure. Some causes of CPTSD are bullying, torture, hunger, homelessness, sleep deprivation and infertility. A 2021 PublicMed Central Study even found 41.3% of infertile women had PTSD symptoms.

Implicit Memory can delay the correlation between exposure to trauma and psychoneuroimmunology. It is the repetitive rehearsing of a routine, activity or verbal response until you can subconsciously mirror the expected results. If an athlete experiences a TBI during a game, their implicit memory would allow them to continue completing rehearsed plays without anyone knowing they experienced a TBI. Wrestler Sam Seitles , during an interview on the

Moving Forward Podcast, explained how he was able to win a wrestling match without any memory of his actions after experiencing a TBI.

Concussions/ Traumatic Brain Injuries are reported in 170,000 to 380,000 sports and recreational activities each year according to the CDC. Since trauma suppresses a person's immune system, research has been conducted to measure the effects of antibiotic use in youth athletes. A ten- year study, 2009-2019, was conducted on over 6,000 youth athletes and there was a relationship between chronic antibiotic use and a reduced risk of concussion.

Tracking the progress of your successes, interests, environment, and overall health assists clinicians with ordering the appropriate tests and prescribing the most effective treatment plans.

Doctor's Visit

Start to gather these items to best prepare for your next doctor's office visit, telehealth call, or ER visit. You can start gathering these items today so that you are not rushed and can avoid forgetting items.

1. Create a box or envelope with the basic items the physician will need to review before they meet with you:
    a. Medical Records
    b. Family Health History
    c. Allergies
    d. Medications
    e. Pharmacy phone number, address
    f. Vitamins
    g. Emergency contact information
    h. List any medical device implants
    i. Drug Allergies
    j. List any previous surgeries
    k. List what you have eaten over the past week

Start to document (write, voice text, draw a picture or video) details about your pain.

2. Location (s)
    a. Size of area
    b. One location or traveling pain
3. Frequency
    a. Repetition or the number of times a day
    b. Time of day (morning, noon, or night)
4. Duration
    a. New pain length
    b. The number of days of the condition
5. Intensity
    a. Sharp pain
    b. Dull pain

~~c. What makes pain worse~~
d. What makes pain go away

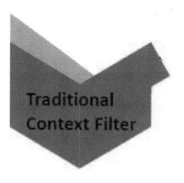

Traditional Context Filters are memories that build a bridge to what's next. Our Innovative ideas must go through these filters. If our goals and purpose are in sync with our personal wants, obstacles become adventurous opportunities.

For example, selling an analog TV with rabbit ears may be hard for an electronics company today. Yet, at one time they were in high demand and most people wanted an analog TV. There were TV manufacturers who experience a lot of success with analog TVs. When the market introduced digital LED TVs, their previous success kept them from embracing change. This type of change could cause them to lose their status.

Analog TV was great during its time. Time does not stand still. We can reference past successes as starting points for our next goal. The key is to celebrate today and set aside time to envision tomorrow.

My Uncle James served our country in Vietnam. He has tons of rich, vivid stories about the social aspects of his tour of duty that would keep you laughing until tears stroll down your face. Everyone loves my Uncle James.

When he greets another serviceman, his face lights up. The instant bond between strangers who have served in the military goes beyond words, categorization, or labeling. Using any one of these items singularly would skew the layers of training and experience that influenced their bond.

My uncle loved his country and is grateful for his opportunity to serve. Still, I never heard him say, "I want to go back to Vietnam."

To ALL servicemen, servicewomen, and veterans, thank you for your service.

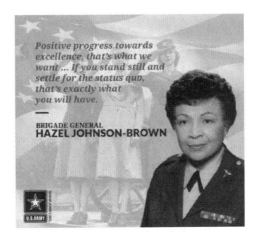

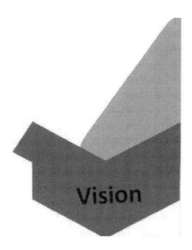

Vision

A vision is something so big that it requires futuristic thought and strategic planning to accomplish. The visionary must make room for new insight that will stretch their self-efficacy. They will experience a continuous desire for something better and believe they can help make it happen.

Kim King, an Emmy Award-winning news reporter, is well known for reporting in-depth stories. Her advocacy delivers a call to action to which her audience has adhered.

Kim's personal story of advocacy was not as clear for local physicians. She had eyelid cancer with visible symptoms. As a news reporter, visibility and appearance are essential for her livelihood and overall self-image. So, she met with several doctors in one practice. She repeatedly asked if it could be cancer because her mother died from cancer. They all concurred with the lead doctor that she had poor makeup-removal skills.

The group of Asheville-referred practitioners had seen many patients with ocular challenges. Friends thought since she was working with the best of the best, she just needed assistance with makeup removal. They dismissed her concerns.

One day, Kim went to another practice that had no affiliation with the previous group of doctors. As soon as the doctor walked into her patient's room, her doctor believed the lump could be cancerous. So, she ordered a biopsy. Within a week, the new doctor confirmed her suspicions: it was cancer.

Kim's goal was total healing. Her goal was a shock to her first group of physicians who thought a visible imperfection was ok. Their difference in expectations inspired Kim to find another pathway to reach her goal.

For some, access to physicians, health literacy, language barriers, and school resources can impede clear receptive language about patient concerns. Researchers from Johns Hopkins University report 40% - 80% of misdiagnoses are due to the failure of medical professionals to take a thorough and comprehensive history from the patient and order the wrong tests. Clearly understand and convey your health norms, and goals, and provide journaled notes on changes to your treatment team at the hospital.

Mental health misdiagnosis ranges from 97.8% for a social anxiety disorder to 65.9% for a major depressive disorder.

Likert Type Scale. This scale is used to measure a person's opinion on a subject. It captures high interest and enjoyment as well as displeasure and indifference.

Clear Thoughts Scale by Kellye Jones

Based on the knowledge I have today....						
	Strongly Agree	Agree	Neutral	Strongly Agree	Disagree	Strongly Disagree
1. I can describe who my vision will help.						
2. I have a personal success story to encourage me.						
3. I completed my daily commitment (time).						
4. I know three people who can provide more Insight.						
5. I understand potential challenges.						
6. I understand how to access resources.						
7. I know my signs of fatigue.						

What one area will I focus on to secure more clarity?

_____

_____

_____

_____

_____

_____

_____

_____

Five action steps to gain clarity

-
-
-
-
-

Chapter Nine:
When Time Management and Availability

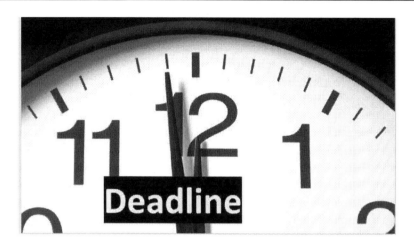

Whether you prefer to complete tasks expeditiously or through procrastination, the key is to finish quality work on time.

Communicating your time management style will help to manage others' expectations and extend your happiness throughout the task. Remember, your team members are counting on YOU to meet your deadlines. Your success is essential for the entire team's win.

Natural benefits for persons who prefer to work expeditiously.

Research and Review. Some people prefer to complete an assignment with the opportunity to make continuous revisions. They enjoy allowing small amounts of time to tweak a document as needed.

Availability for others. Time to help others.

Acknowledgment. Praise from teachers and bragging rights.

Leadership. It subtly establishes a person as a credible leader to onlookers.

Feedback. Teacher response, guidance on corrections.

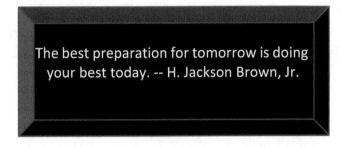

The best preparation for tomorrow is doing your best today. -- H. Jackson Brown, Jr.

Natural benefits for persons who prefer to work on completing projects closer to their deadlines.

Optimist. Others may think they are not working, while they are strategically planning a process. Self-aware.

Inclusive. They are empaths who want to help the largest number of people.

Crowd Control. Commotion can be stressful. They may wait for the crowd to dissipate.

Thrill seekers. They enjoy the challenge of racing to finish. Good stress excites and enhances engagement.

Let the fun begin.

Availability

"Hi, I did not want to interrupt you, but I need help with one small item. Let me know when you have a few free minutes." How many times a day are you asked this question, or do you ask others this question?

Empaths will often say yes to multiple requests because they do not want to disappoint others.

There are two common types of empath responses.

Affective empathy enables a person to feel the joy and pain of a person while they are communicating. They will laugh with you, not at you, and even shed tears with you. They are emotionally invested in you.

Cognitive empathy enables a deeper understanding of how "if-then" responses will impact the speaker.

Example. If someone states they are having a bad hair day, a person with cognitive empathy would understand showing them pictures of beautiful hair models may not make them feel better. The comparison or an inability to reach the perfect hairstyle is what made the person feel like they were having a bad day. A person with cognitive empathy will avoid responses that devalue others. They will seek responses that empower others.

Making room for self-empathy helps round out your emotions. It ensures you are refueling yourself. Develop a timetable, progress checks, and a deadline for accomplishing personal goals. It is not selfish- it is self-preservation to see joy, fulfillment, and peace for **yourself.** It's really ok to smile and embrace steps of elevation in your own life.

When flight attendants provide safety instructions to passengers, they tell passengers, "In case of emergency, place your mask on you first." Too often, some people place their satisfaction as least important. They begin to blend helping everyone else get ahead and stay stagnant or move further away from their dreams because they forget to incorporate a time for doing what brings them joy. Invest time in what refuels **YOU** - a nap, a gym workout, trip to the museum, a social gathering filled with laughter or a combination of activities. As you evolve some of your core interests may still bring you the most joy, so try to incorporate them. Making a plan to do what you enjoy, putting the mask on yourself to breath first, is not selfish; it is self-preservation. Enjoy it. Joy is a solid foundation for greater effectiveness, efficiency, and energy in accomplishing your goals.

The Empathy Test Link and Two Time Management Test Links are included in the Reference Section.

What are your established availability assistance hours?

What do you believe you will be able to better accomplish by reducing your hours of availability?

_____
_____
_____
_____
_____
_____

How will you hold yourself accountable for keeping these hours?

_____
_____
_____
_____
_____
_____

Chapter Ten:
Where I Am Ready to Go

Our social and physical environment can unknowingly challenge phobias such as blue light, an aversion to or avoidance of light; claustrophobia extreme or irrational fear of small, enclosed spaces; allodynia the extreme pain felt from touch and even a sticker nametag; and trypophobia, the feeling of disgust or fear when you see patterns with lots of holes.

Some stimuli will elicit strong likes, and we want more similar experiences. Unfavorable environmental catalysts stir strong feelings of dislike, and we will avoid them in the future.

Periodically, our list of like and dislike items shifts because of our cultural competence. This is the ability to develop relationships with people whose culture is different from our own. This is not about dominance, influence, or assimilation to maintain a harmonious environment. It is about respect and appreciation of diverse beliefs and traditions.

The challenge with adhering to traditional norms instead of cultural competence is the demographics of neighborhoods, workplaces, and schools are continuously evolving. More diverse people are attending school together, working in one setting, and attending the same conferences. Different interests, skills, resources, and pursuits in the community, make it harder to compartmentalize another person's interest. The key to successful engagement, mutual interest, and sustainable relationships is remembering, one size can no longer fit all.

Our traditional filters might have us think we know what should work best for others. These assumptions can lead to disappointment, disengagement, stress, and just an overall dimming of joy. Think of Goldilocks. Her story begins, "Once upon a time, there was a little girl named Goldilocks." The average-year- old cub weighs 80 lbs. The average weight of a 10-year-old girl is 55 lbs. Goldilocks is now tired and ready to take a nap. She is trying to figure out where to sleep. The baby bear slept in a bed that Goldilocks could easily fit in. It may seem like that is where she would be happiest, but she was not.

Assumptions could lead a reader to believe that the baby bear's bed would be the best bed for Goldilocks. Conversely, Goldilocks thought it was too soft. She tried all of the beds. You know you better than anyone else what you enjoy. She did not settle on where she would sleep until she found the place which best suited her needs.

We should all have some Goldilocks characteristics in us. It's ok to measure your success in different social settings with different environmental stimuli. Some people may enjoy studying at the library while others will enjoy their room or the kitchen table with background conversations. Differentiating sounds and images which motivate you or stir creative thought, put you to sleep, or pull you away from your work for hours is key. When you explore your options, you will be able to more effectively communicate why an environment works. When you travel to new locations, you will have an easier time replicating things you need to succeed.

Understanding her needs and a willingness to go beyond complacency helped Goldilocks to enjoy her rest. Later on, it gave her the energy to run away from the bears.

Some preferences are less obvious until we start to dig deeper and ask more questions. Here are the links to a few reference quizzes.

Sensory Intelligence Quiz, Claustrophobia Test, Trypophobia Quiz

One day, Kim started to get irritated and barged out of the room when another coworker started eating. Watching and hearing Kim's daily frustration and complaints of headaches, I asked, "What is wrong?" Kim explained how she felt our coworker was insensitive to everyone in the breakroom.

She chews on her popcorn so loudly until I cannot think." The next day, I watched and listened for the loud chewing. I did not hear it. No one else seemed to be bothered by our coworkers' chewing.

The next day, after seeing Kim's anger again, I asked if her headaches were getting progressively worse or constant. She said, "They spiked up and became unbearable. She makes me so angry." I then explained misophonia to her: irritability, anger, and headaches can arise from a repetitive sound. The pitch and volume do not matter. It is like a sensory processing order – a condition that affects how your brain processes audio stimuli -- with aggression.

It's easier to find coping solutions, alter environments, and avoid settings when you understand the core of a challenge.

Discovering and enjoying awe-inspiring experiences helps our social and emotional well-being.

Spending time in a place with fond memories can release dopamine and endorphins. Arriving at that place can provide an instant rush and elicit vivid details from past events. A Harvard study found a person's joy has a greater impact on social skills and interpersonal relationships than their genes.

Where is the place that makes you smile and gives you a thrill? Is it outdoors, an art museum, or a dance theater? Some examples are nature, an art museum, an amusement park, or the beach. Take time to think about your visit to one of your favorite places. Note details on what made that experience memorable. Can you recreate a similar experience or make revisiting that place one of your goals?

Typically, things or places that stimulate your five senses are places of awe. Where is that place?

Growing up, at least once a month, my dad and I would travel to his office in Manhattan. After he finished his paperwork, we would order hot dogs at Nathan's in Times Square. Then we would sit at the counter for hours watching diverse groups of people walk by and discuss our plans to help humanity. Before heading home, we would walk for at least four more hours.

Our walk would be about embracing the amazing eclectic vibes of Manhattan. From the chants of the Hare Krishnas to the street dancers and subway dancers to the powerful artwork in the Village to price haggling with street vendors for sunglasses or gloves, watching the tourist amazement of the Times Square lights there was tons of excitement. We always found beauty and gifts in the things we saw. The Hare Krishnas' togetherness and joy of inclusion were evident as onlookers inquired about their religion. Such a memory cannot be taken away regardless of the challenges and disappointments they may face in attempting to educate others. There were street hagglers who made the act of negotiation an art. My dad and I would stand over to the side and watch them teach their apprentice the art of vending.

Our day would end with purchasing an appetizer from a restaurant in Chinatown and a dessert from a restaurant in Little Italy. We had to take home a treasure to my mom. Our walks and talks were all so beautiful because of the eclectic energy. There was an influx of new tourists, people from different socioeconomic groups talking together at one table, and more harmony. It all kept us engaged, amazed, enriched, and excited about the ever-changing and welcoming environment around us.

Our Saturday trips were more than a visit to his office, attending a professional sports game, or getting Nathan's hot dog. They were times of familial discovery. Daddy shared contrasting stories about his life as a tobacco farmer and a New York City businessman.

There were contrasts that addressed all modes of environmental stimuli – sight, sound, smell, and touch. We would talk about the rich, beautiful scents of the farmer's greenery as we walked past the hot pretzel stand and the vibrant fresh scents of a street vendor's Brazilian Nuts'. There were fun stories where you could envision the warm embrace of family members during

Sunday dinners as we walked past couples holding hands and smiling. He would tell of the beautiful, peaceful nights with the sweet sounds of nature as we walked past the loud sounds of honking horns and street musicians. Both environments were full of alluring traits. We spent many holidays at his childhood home, which had outdoor plumbing, so I already knew the difference. Still, it was so amazing to hear about the South in my dad's own words.

The one thing my dad hated was pre-judging others. He would say, "When you take the limits off, you will see greatness all around you. Then research the magnificence and future positive implications of what you just learned." Stereotypes could have kept him fighting a country boy label and proving himself to others repeatedly in a big city.

My dad loved his company. They embraced and promoted him even with his very different culture. Our trips to Manhattan and continuous exposure to eclectic audiences were to make sure I avoided stereotypes and saw the best in all people.

Think excellence and you will see excellence.

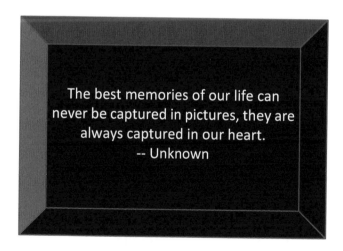

Social Settings and Personality Types

Even though I love diverse audiences and won my high school Senior Class Superlative "Most Talkative," I am not an extrovert. I am an ambivert. This seemed strange until I heard Oprah say, "I am an introvert with extrovert tendencies."

Finally, more people have the opportunity to prefer more than two extreme social settings. Understanding the differences between the four can assist a person with stating what they need. It's ok to say, this large gathering is draining me emotionally and I need a break. This is normal and to be expected for three of the four personality types. Clearly communicating your needs will help to manage the expectations of others and give you more peace.

Do crowds energize you?

Is quiet time by yourself, in your house a necessity to process your thoughts?

Anticipation of an unwanted social setting can arouse negative nervous excitement or fear. Anticipation of a favorable social setting can arouse positive nervous excitement or eustress.

It is the same emotion of excitement with polarized reference frames.

Take time to find your method of escape when you are in a less comfortable social setting.

Let's find your favorite social setting and personality type.

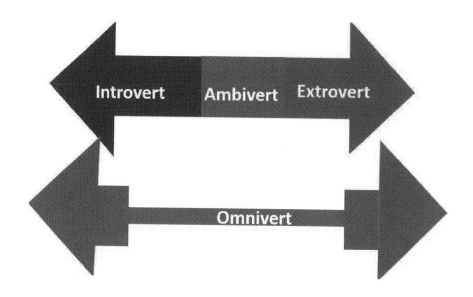

Social Behaviors

Confirmation bias and exposure limitations can lead to a finite scope of your gifts. **All** social personalities make forward-thinking teams better. The more you understand about your strengths, the better you will be able to advance your self-image.

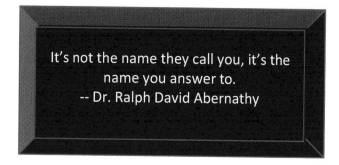

Ambiverts

Persons who are mistakenly viewed as Bipolar

Ambiverts enjoy one-to-one and smaller group conversations where there is more subject matter depth. Their social traits of extraversion and introversion help them to have individual talks with a wide range of personalities. More than half of our population can be classified as ambiverts.

Ambiverts are able to adapt to the room, communicate creative next-step thoughts, and stay current. Overall, they are balanced leaders embracing assertiveness, empathy, listening, problem-solving, and discernment of the bigger picture.

An ambivert's flexibility can cause indecisiveness. If there are two or more great social options for the day, it may take an ambivert longer to decide which option to choose.

Ambiverts are often misunderstood by onlookers who are only familiar with extroverts and introverts. Some, even loved ones, may think an ambivert is moody or even bipolar. Ambiverts have situational or temporary challenges where they bounce back quickly. Persons with bipolar socio-occupational (social and work) activities are impacted over a long period of time by their moodiness.

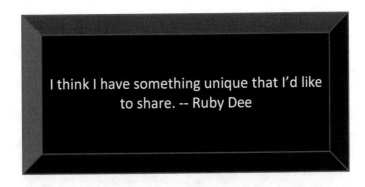

I think I have something unique that I'd like to share. -- Ruby Dee

Introverts

Persons who may be viewed as suffering from depression Introverts recharge in physical or mental isolation, where they can more clearly analyze and process their thoughts. They typically have a small group of friends. Even though they prefer to take mental or physical breaks from the crowd, when they are in a crowd, they observe and absorb lots of information about their environment. They listen attentively to others.

Processing the many details of various conversations can become overwhelming, so they may seek mental or physical breaks from the crowd. Oprah Winfrey has stated she spends time in the bathroom in social settings to take a breather from the crowd.

There are five types of introverts.

1. Social Introverts prefer smaller group settings or time alone. This preference has been confused with social anxiety, which is fear.

2. Thinking Introverts prefer to study and research subject matters. During an in-depth topic discussion, they may gaze away in silence to process new information.

3. Anxious Introverts can be afraid of social environments and strive to avoid social settings to protect their peace.

4. Restrained Introverts prefer routines and predictability. They are introspective, and reflective, and may appear unemotional.

5. Forced introverts are a blend of introverts and loners. Introverts and loners are different. Introverts enjoy small groups of people whereas loners avoid people. Forced Introverts feel rejected by their environment, so they stay to themselves.

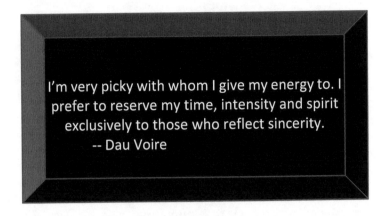

> I'm very picky with whom I give my energy to. I prefer to reserve my time, intensity and spirit exclusively to those who reflect sincerity.
> -- Dau Voire

Extroverts

Persons who are confused with Historic Personality Disorder (HPD)

Extroverts enjoy social events. They have larger-than-life personalities that can make them the life of the party.

At the same time, their enthusiasm can be snubbed in a more reserved crowd. This response causes crowd-pleasing extroverts to feel lonely, develop low self-esteem, and need peer affirmation. It is the starved extrovert/forced introvert scenario mentioned above.

There are two types of extroverts.

1. Agentic Extroverts are go-getters who excel in engagement and leadership. The donkey in *Shrek* talks a lot, has high energy, and is the center of attention in many movie scenes. Donkey is an agentic extrovert.

2. Affiliative Extroverts are friendly, affirming, and inclusive. The main character in Ferris Bueller's Day Off is charming, adventurous, and an affiliative extrovert.

Research studies have identified advanced cerebral activity in extroverts. So, asking an extrovert to change is like asking them to rewire their brain.

Omniverts

Persons who are mistakenly thought to have Dual Personality Disorder. (DPD)

Omniverts have the gift of residing in the middle of the extremes of an outgoing extrovert and a shy introvert. Their adaptability to their surroundings can make them seem untiring, but in reality, the back and forth is mentally exhausting for them. Balancing social expectations can cause anxiety, depression, and low self-esteem as they seek to fulfill other's needs and ignore their own.

This goes back to confirmation bias. If a person meets an omnivert in their outgoing extrovert stage, this person might expect the omnivert to always be in extrovert mode. If they try to explain their fatigue, they may be faced with comments like, "You cannot be tired. You have lots of energy.' or "What's wrong? You seem depressed."

Onlookers can be quick to judge because they are just looking to solve a problem. If you are aware of your social needs, you can inform others immediately to avoid defending yourself later. Friends will understand how to support you and help you get the rest you need to keep your superstar light shining bright.

Omniverts who prioritize "me time" enable themselves to unwind and recharge for their next adventure.

Omniverts have a broad grasp of networking. They socialize like extroverts. Their introverted strengths enable them to use discernment and listen intuitively when capturing conversation details. They are highly sought-after problem-solvers.

Problem solvers.

Persons unfamiliar with the unique talents of an omnivert may misconstrue their chameleon personality, availability, and understanding of diverse audiences as unpredictable. This perception is even tougher in environments that require conformity and adherence to tradition.

> Some people don't understand that sitting in your own house in peace, eating snacks and minding your business is priceless....
> -- Fb/lessonslearnedinlifeinc

Chapter Eleven:
Why -The Big Picture

"Why" people enjoy analyzing a subject to get to the core of the challenge. They uncover breakthrough solutions to circumvent and disrupt repetitive, systemic, or network challenges. They are big-picture people who thrive with eclectic collaborative thought because their focus is depth, longevity, and sustainability. Some may say they are dreamers and explorers because they focus on the intangible and unseen. They are visionaries working for innovation and evolution.

They are the paradigm shift people who enjoy coloring outside of the lines.

Walt Disney enjoyed creating an escape through his drawings. From an early age, he practiced several forms of drawing and became a cartoonist. While serving as a Red Cross ambulance driver, he painted cartoon characters on the outside of ambulances. He wanted to create happiness wherever he went.

After his time overseas, he created Oswald the Lucky Rabbit with Ubbe Ert Iwwerks, known as Ub Iwerks for Universal Studios. Disney wanted a character that audiences would love, and Universal wanted slapstick humor. The studio moved forward with Disney's choice, and audiences loved Oswald. Oswald was a success.

After seeing such great success, Disney scheduled a meeting with its executives in New York to ask for a raise. "Film producer [Charles] Mintz, tired of Walt's demands and in disbelief of his actual talent, began negotiating for more Oswald shorts without Walt."

When Disney arrived in New York, Mintz fired him. Disney's termination caused Disney to have a nervous breakdown. He spent time away from animation.

Ultimately, his desire to create happiness wherever pushed him out of his sadness. His skills and interest gave him a renewed sense of purpose. Disney continued pursuing an even greater imagination with a desire to make dreams come true. He created the 500 acres of Disneyland Amusement Park just seven miles away from America's first amusement park, 57 acres of Knotts Berry Farm Amusement Park. Later, with the hope of creating a futuristic, always ahead-of-the-times facility that would stir others to imagine, he envisioned Epcot.

> If your plan is for one year, plant rice. If your plan is for ten years, plant trees. If your plan is for one hundred years, educate children.
> -- Confucius

He then began to build Disney World. It is a place with infinite possibilities for future dreamers.

The work of "Why" people is entailed in their ability to influence innovative, long-term, infinite, and futuristic vision. For those who think of short-term goals, the thought processes of "Why" people can be challenging to quantify. If you are a forward-thinking person, keep going. You may be the founder of our next theme park.

Dream Big.

Let's Learn More about Your Personality Strengths

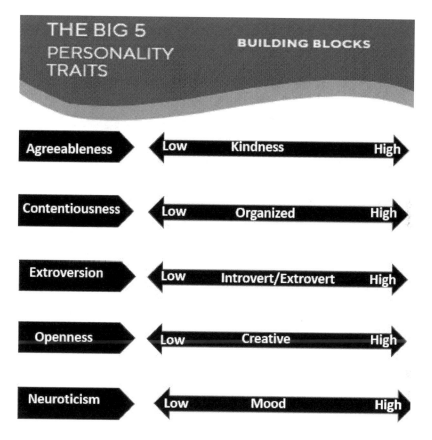

Gordon Allport uncovered 4,504 adjectives that describe personality traits in his search for personality adjectives. Many years and philosophers later, Lewis Goldberg discovered that these words fit into five categories.

The five categories are Openness, Conscientiousness, Extraversion, Agreeableness, and Neuroticism. They are called the "Big 5." The Big 5 assessment provides insight into a person's high or low preference for a trait.

The Big Five Assessment

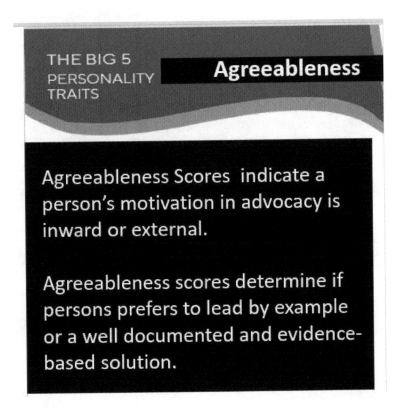

    Altruism is a predominant characteristic in agreeable persons.

    On many Sunday mornings, my family and I watched Feed the Children on TV. Shortly following the show, my 10-year-old daughter walked into the kitchen to talk to her father and me. At first, she made small talk. Then she said, "I want to talk about something fundamental to me." There was silence in the room. She continued, "This year, I do not want any presents for Christmas. Instead, I would like you to send the money you spend on my gifts to a little boy in Africa. Can we please pay for the meals of a little boy from Africa on *Feed the*

Children? I will not ask for any gifts later because this is something I want."

To this day, my daughter is incredibly giving to her friends.

There is also contextual altruism. Specific scenarios evoke more intense emotions, creating a selfless response.

My son Noah has PANS/ PANDAS, and he is a nonverbal eloper. Persons with PANS/PANADAS and autism elope. Actually, 49% of persons with autism who elope, or flee from a safe environment, he has sat still for very few things in life.

One stereotypical characteristic of the two diagnoses is alexithymia – an inability to be aware of, explicitly identify, or describe one's feelings -- but I, like most parents of children with autism and PANS/PANDAS, can provide instances that suggest all persons with autism should not be deemed unempathetic.

My parents raised me to be the best Kellye that I can be. Our family motto was "Only compete with your last best effort, and you will always grow.". This standard presented some highs and some lows. The lows, I managed with no more than a day to cry, talk, and eat it out; then it was back to business. When I would cry it out, if my son Noah saw me, he would sit beside me and wipe my tears. As soon as I stopped crying, he was off and running again.

Understanding this characteristic, especially contextually, could enable greater sensitization and understanding when pauses or rest breaks may help make your communication more productive.

THE BIG 5 PERSONALITY TRAITS — Conscientiousness

Conscientiousness Scores indicate how a persons will organize their thoughts and work space.

Using your best-suited style will help with timely goal achievement

Conversely, using a nonpreferred style will increase dependency and delays.

There was a TV show called *The Odd Couple* that featured two roommates with polarized approaches to solving problems. In the end, it was the interdependency of their personality traits that brought forth the best solution.

Your uniqueness is needed because YOU are awesome.

> **THE BIG 5 PERSONALITY TRAITS**
>
> **Extroversion**
>
> Extroversion Scores indicate a persons need for external stimuli.
>
> An extroverts brain has more dopamine. They are less aroused to it so they need more to fulfill a natural need.
>
> Introverts have less so a little dopamine is fine.

Understanding your character strengths can assist you in finding the best frequency, duration, and intensity of social engagement to feel fulfilled. If you should experience lulls, reflect on the attributes of a fun time. It can be easier to replicate the attributes than the event.

Example. If you enjoy watching movies and talking about the scenes in real-time with friends, going to the movie theater without friends may not provide the same sense of social joy. Maybe calling friends and family and watching a movie simultaneously while talking about the movie scenes in real-time would be more rewarding.

Following your unique interests will help you bypass voids and feel more accomplished. There will be detours, and dead ends on the journey but stay with it. Face new challenges with temperance, and hope. Success is closer than you think.

> Without dopamine, desire died. And without desire, action stopped. -- James Clear (*Atomic Habits*)

THE BIG 5 PERSONALITY TRAITS

Openness

Openness scores indicate your views on change and variety.

More open people are curious. They enjoy engaging new people and enjoying new places.

Less open minded people prefer to tradition and organized schedules. They prefer a few specific interests

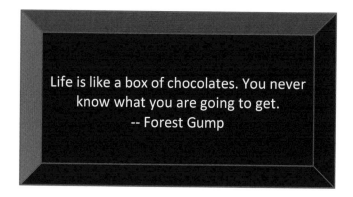

Life is like a box of chocolates. You never know what you are going to get.
-- Forest Gump

When I asked former NBA Player John Wallace what the key to his success was, he replied, "Consistency." He practiced shooting a basketball for hours a day every day. He did not care about the weather; rain or shine, he played every day.

John said, "If a girl wanted to date me, our dates had to be at the basketball court." They would retrieve basketballs for him while he practiced free throws.

John had other social options, but he was not open to anything that kept him from practicing.

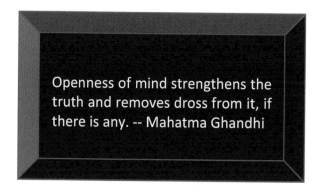

Openness of mind strengthens the truth and removes dross from it, if there is any. -- Mahatma Ghandhi

THE BIG 5 PERSONALITY TRAITS

Neuroticism

Neuroticism scores indicate a persons tolerance for environmental stimuli or a peripheral nerve disorder (hyperesthesia)

When a person is overstimulated frustration can cause aggression such as misophonia.

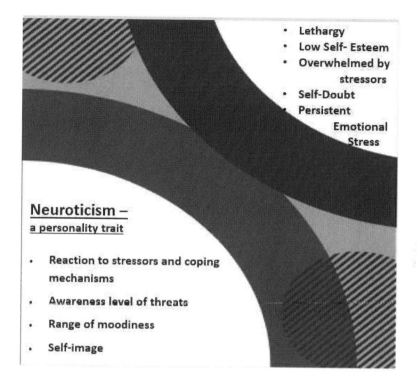

Neuroticism addresses how you will respond to situational stressors. Persons with high neuroticism have habituated to fewer sudden, surprise stressors.

For example, the first time you hear a school fire alarm, a rush of nervousness may cause you to lose your train of thought. After several fire drills, persons with a low level of neuroticism have habituated to the sound and will casually line up and get ready to exit the school. Persons with higher neuroticism who have not habituated to the sound will experience a maintained level of fear. Developing your preferred coping mechanism to address alarming sounds will enable you to shorten the period of overstimulation.

Neurosis and psychosis are different. Neurosis is the constant questioning of self-worth and self-efficacy. Psychosis consists of debilitating thoughts that reduce engagement with others and surroundings.

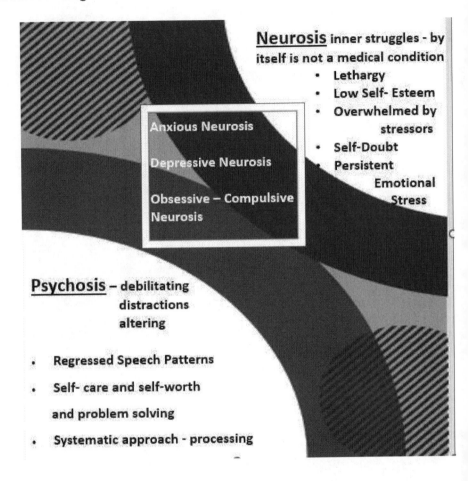

Neurosis inner struggles - by itself is not a medical condition
- Lethargy
- Low Self- Esteem
- Overwhelmed by stressors
- Self-Doubt
- Persistent Emotional Stress

Anxious Neurosis

Depressive Neurosis

Obsessive – Compulsive Neurosis

Psychosis – debilitating distractions altering

- Regressed Speech Patterns
- Self- care and self-worth and problem solving
- Systematic approach - processing

The HEXACO Personality Inventory Assessment

HEXACO

HERARCHY OF
SELF-INTEREST

- **Agreeableness**
- **Conscientiousness**
- **Emotionality**
- **Extroversion**
- **Emotionality**
- **Open to Experience**
- **Honesty - Humility**

  HEXACO provides Likert scale insight on six personality traits. It is similar to the Big 5 assessment with one additional category: Honesty-Humility. Honesty-humility scores inform individuals of their underlying self-interest when pursuing a result. Are they situationally honest because the end result will be in their own best interest? Or does your prioritization of honesty- humility extend to self-sacrifice and avoidance of shortcuts?

During the recent global pandemic, there was almost no toilet paper in many local stores. Many days, there was none on the shelf. At the same time, I saw Facebook postings of persons with closets full of toilet paper. A person with lower scores in Honesty-Humility would think of self-preservation before integrity.

Shortly after, the local stores posted "toilet paper purchase limit" signs in front of the toilet paper displays. How would the postings impact a person with high honesty-humility scores versus a person with low honesty-humility scores? What is the critical honesty-humility limitation for the crystallization of your vision?

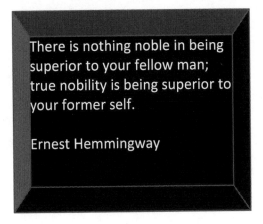

There is nothing noble in being superior to your fellow man; true nobility is being superior to your former self.

Ernest Hemmingway

There is a HEXACO Assessment link in the Reference Section

Chapter Twelve:
How - The Details

"How" people enjoy managing the logistical process of meeting daily tangible goals. Their ability to drill down on details enables them to correct routine flaws.

They prefer daily routines, advance notice, and planning before introducing a new idea. Their in-depth analysis and creation of systems provides a more solid foundation.

As a child, Thomas Edison had challenges keeping up with his peers academically. One day, administrators at his school expelled Edison, stating there was no hope for him.

Edison's mother told him he was a genius. She fibbed and told him the letter from the school stated he was too smart and should be schooled at home. As a teacher, I can imagine his lessons entailed a lot of attention to detail and repetition.

Today, Thomas Edison is known for inventing the incandescent light bulb, phonograph, motion picture camera, and improving the telegraph, and the telephone.

Chapter Thirteen:
"Why" People and "How" People

The story of Walt Disney exemplifies the different ways "how" and "why" people measure effectiveness.

In the Walt Disney story, Disney was looking to have his audience develop a lasting admiration for Oswald. He wanted audiences to tune in to watch a persona develop. There would be an infinite number of possibilities for the character to connect with audiences. Disney's success would be based on an evolution of thought and kindness.

It may take years to see the full maturation of a "why" person's work because their work is so big until all of the moving pieces have to align before the evolution, innovation, and paradigm shift take place. This type of change requires

1. Creative Thought to imagine and map out sequential steps
2. Collaboration. Disney had several persons help him purchase the land for Disney World.
3. Commitment. Change is harder for some decision-makers. Listen to your opposition then begin to educate them. You will have to educate and reeducate them to support your idea of change.
4. Courage. Fortitude to move forward despite the obstacles in front of you will help you maintain momentum. Momentum invites excitement. Excitement supports longevity.

Universal's Charles Mintz had a "How" people approach success. "How" people manage the details of people's performance, tasks, inventory, and processes. Mintz wanted to duplicate the current tangible and immediate gratification humor format of favored programs where measurement is easily defined, and funding is less risky. It was challenging for Mintz to validate or appreciate Disney's visionary approach, which Mintz found so contrary to his core values that he eventually fired Disney.

"Why" people have a mindset of infinitive evolution and the ability to stay ahead of the curve. "How" people have an infinite set of pathways to sell tangible products- vacations, insurance, computers, and more.

Understanding personality traits elevates trust, validation, and excitement. Knowing your unique strengths encourages engagement and skilled contributions. The internet has provided more business owners access to global customers with distinct communication and validation norm tests.

Oprah's final show comment, "I've talked to nearly 30,000 people on this show, and all 30,000 had one thing in common: They all wanted validation. If I could reach through this television and sit on your sofa or sit on a stool in your kitchen right now, I would tell you that every single person you will ever meet shares that common desire. They want to know: 'Do you see me? Do you hear me? Does what I say mean anything to you?' "

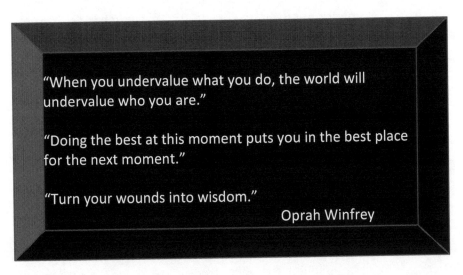

"When you undervalue what you do, the world will undervalue who you are."

"Doing the best at this moment puts you in the best place for the next moment."

"Turn your wounds into wisdom."

Oprah Winfrey

How and Why Messaging

The show Undercover Boss highlighted the vast difference goals and duties of a visionary, big picture Chief Executive Officers (Why People) and the task efficiency oriented of front-line employees (How People). Schools have Principles (Why People) and Administrators (How People). Sports teams have owners (Why People) and Operations Managers (How People). Both are essential for operational success and customer/ employee/ team/ student satisfaction. They have unique missions which need to be communicated to a larger audience.

How messaging helps viewers understand the tactical, logistical, and sequential components of a task or activity– employee training manuals, directions for use, and warning labels.

While working in the hospitality industry at very upscale hotel, the hotel manager began to emphasize the need to "put heads in beds" during the weekends. The hotel's occupancy was running about 50% most weekends and he wanted to fill it up. So, we added sports groups and more with four plus occupants per room. Our hotel was not ready for the high demand for towels, late pool hours with attendants, high demand for the hotel shuttle and more.

From the first thirty minutes of guest check-ins until weeks after the last checkout, disgruntled guests voiced their complaints. The negative comment card feedback came from weekend sports team guests, long-term and month-long corporate guests who were not used to the high-volume weekend activity. Over extended employees also expressed their frustrations about staffing shortages. The gaps in communication and expectations between senior staff, staff and guests led to many refunds and complimentary offers for future stays to large groups of people.

After these challenges, our hotel's human resources department added more operations training modules, to our existing manual, on how to manage large groups with quadruple plus occupancy. A misinterpretation of procedures and short cuts can lead to huge setbacks.

On average, customers will share good experiences with nine people and bad experiences with 16 people. Then add social media with call to action messaging on social media and via text, and subsequent conversations.

Why messaging creates the future need and stronger desire for consumers to purchase products and services. Marketing, outreach, communications specialists, public relations personnel, and reputation repair strategists are hired to create and convey this ever-evolving message through relational and transactional sales and marketing. Culture and climate trends dictate the longevity and impact of a message.

Many top retailers have large budgets for marketing and promotions.
1. Budweiser, with the 2022 best selling beer Bud Light, has spent over $500 million on Super Bowl commercials. A 2023 Budweiser ad was not well received by consumer consequently sales were adversely impacted.
2. In 2022, Amazon spent almost $13.5 billion US dollars on advertising and Walmart spent $3.4 billion on advertising in the US.
3. In 2020, during COVID, McDonald's spent $702 million on advertising and promotions
4. In 2022, Burger King boosted its measured media advertising expenditure in the United States to almost 500 million dollars in 2022, up from 326 million dollars in 2021.

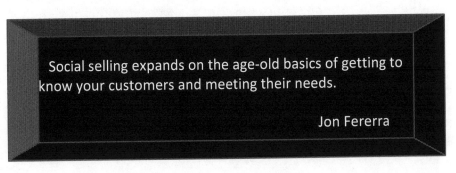

> Social selling expands on the age-old basics of getting to know your customers and meeting their needs.
>
> Jon Fererra

Effective messaging is essential for industry leaders to stay ahead of the game. Xerox Alto was the first large scale personal computer (PC). It was produced almost 10 years prior to market competition and the smaller digital PC. Xerox became very comfortable, fixed, with its profit margins and traditions. They had advanced technology and salesmen, but they were missing the component which builds brand loyalty – marketing research and analysis. Sometimes sales, marketing and communications are viewed as one and the same, but they are three completely different approaches to messaging. Today, many consumers may not be aware of XEROX's innovation due to the absence of prioritize marketing.

As successful "How" and "Why" people hone in on their unique skills and interest they also remember to include messaging in their plan of action.

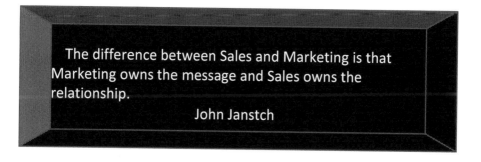

The difference between Sales and Marketing is that Marketing owns the message and Sales owns the relationship.
John Janstch

Chapter Fourteen:
VARK and Multi-Intellectual

Around age 2, my son Jay's doctor diagnosed him with audio processing delay. We read articles, talked to other clinicians, and worked side-by-side with caregivers to learn more about the diagnosis. Over and over, we heard two words of advice

1. Sound out your words
2. Use picture exchange cards.

As an out-of-the-box thinker, my mom and I decided to add Sing-A-Long videos to those two strategies. After watching the videos a few times, we would reduce the volume. By the end of 30 to 40 days, Jay would read the videos with no sound.

Fast forward to ten years later. As we were getting ready to leave the house, I turned to Jay and said, "Go get your shirt." He leaped up and ran to the door with his Magna Doodle writing pad. Then I stated, "Jay, we cannot leave until you get your shirt. Please go get your shirt." Jay just stood at the door. I walked over to Jay and looked him in the face because he reads lips. I said, "What did Mommy say?" He then wrote C H U R C H. He thought I said church not shirt.

He is an audio learner. Classical music helps him focus. His dominant audio-learning style relies heavily on intonation and supplemental writing. The four more common expressive and receptive language styles are visual, audio, written, and kinetic (VARK). Understanding your style will help you help others clarify information the way you like to learn. This type of clarity will provide you with an advantage and more fulfilling conversations.

Jay's interests were science and math. I would incorporate language with math to help him retain new words. The Multi-Intellectual assessment can help with discovering areas of mastery, interest, and analogies.

Expressive and Receptive Language A link for this quiz is located in the Reference section.

Communication has two fundamental functions. They are expressive language and receptive language.

Expressive language is the speaker's interpretation of
1. what the receiver will need to clearly understand their message and respond appropriately
2. the skills and resources needed to effectively present their message
3. a successful message delivery

Receptive language is the listener's interpretation of
1. the speaker's message
2. how the speaker wants them to respond.

Similar life experiences, culture, dialect, geography, and more can enhance the fluidity of this communication and help the speaker receive their preferred response. Variances in historical experiences, individual goals, scarcity, and competition can skew intentions and clarity. The greatest challenge with speakers having diverse frames of reference is quite often listeners do not have the time to figure out the speaker's intentions.

Incorporating the four VARK (visual, audio, written, and kinetic) communication styles can help increase the clarity of your message. VARK equips teachers, trainers, leaders, and more with the agility to address a larger and more diverse audience in one setting.

Expressive and Receptive Language

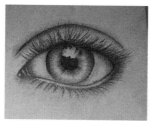

Items that visual communicators may prefer:
- Charts and graphs for comparative analysis and spatial organization.
- Videos for a more in-depth understanding of context.
- Pictures for the implementation process.

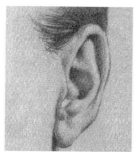

Items that audio communicators may prefer:
- Record yourself explaining the features and benefits of a topic
- Have listeners close their eyes as you provide the descriptive details of sounds.
- Add classical music to a PowerPoint presentation.
- Conversations - chats, discussions, lectures, Stories

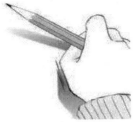

Items that written communicators may prefer:
- Provide space for linear notetaking
- Provide non-linear fillable note-taking options such as mapping, charting, and graphing to help with spatial organization.

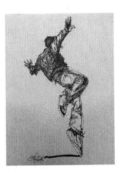

Items that kinetic communicators may prefer:
- Use objects with texture to introduce contrast or shifts to conceptual explanations.
- Provide manipulatives to build or dissect a concept physically. It empowers by providing control of the pace of model development and understanding.

Chapter Fifteen:
Assess, Advance, and Stay Agile

Moving forward requires going through unfamiliar and possibly unchartered territory.

Atychiphobia --fear of failure -- along your journey can hinder planning, progress, and prosperity. To go beyond this stage, take small steps to stay on track for success. Like Goldilocks, keep sampling until you find the pace best for you.

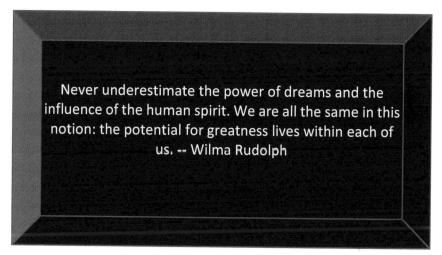

> Never underestimate the power of dreams and the influence of the human spirit. We are all the same in this notion: the potential for greatness lives within each of us. -- Wilma Rudolph

Five hundred years ago, Michel de Montaigne said: "My life has been filled with terrible misfortune; most of which never happened." We can break this 500-year-old habit with more self-compassion.

> I want to be remembered as one who tried.
> -- Dorothy Height

Assess Your Wheelhouse. Make sure you are filtering in uplifting feedback daily or as often as possible. If you are continually affirming others but not receiving affirmation in your love language you can experience burnout. Mutual affirmations are always great.

Reciprocity and imbibing support can come naturally or by request. Some people may not realize there is a void because you have not expressed your affirmation needs. Understand what type of responses you want and need to feel valued and maintain balance.

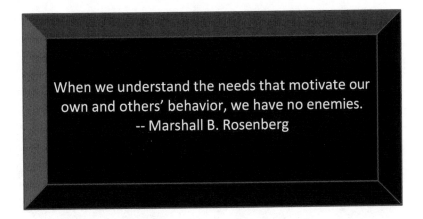

When we understand the needs that motivate our own and others' behavior, we have no enemies.
-- Marshall B. Rosenberg

The Five Love Languages of expression are

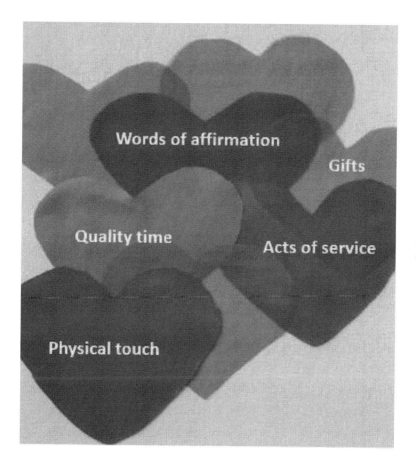

A National Institute of Health research study led by Daniel K. Campbell- Meiklejohn revealed "The opinions of others alter a fundamental function of the brain's ventral striatum response allowing room for a long-term change of values." Whether or not we have long conversations with others or practice onlooking, we take in items which influence how we will engage with others. It starts in infancy and continues throughout our lives.

Sometimes we will learn things that could make our lives easier. Other times, we know things we want to avoid like the plague.

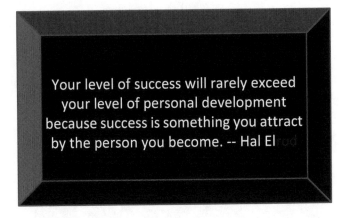

> Your level of success will rarely exceed your level of personal development because success is something you attract by the person you become. -- Hal Elrod

The assumption that tradition is the best and only route to success reminds me of David seeking to fight Goliath wearing Saul's battle gear. Saul viewed his armor as a needed asset in battle. Wearing it affirmed his strength as a leader. Since he was the king, why did he not put it on, feel affirmed, and go fight Goliath? There has to be something deeper than the suit of armor to provide him with the confidence to fight or not fight. Saul was a crowd-pleaser. He sought words of affirmation. The crowds talk about the size of Goliath led Saul into hiding and even sending a child to fight his battle for him.

Saul mistakenly believed his strength came from a uniform, so he encouraged the little boy David to wear it. David was humble enough to try Saul's suggestion. It did not work for David.

Our expectations and hope are derived, in art, from our love language. Words of encouragement helped Saul fight other battles and win. Words of praise for others led Saul into jealous and violent rages.

Knowing your love language can help you manage your social circles, messaging intake, and appreciation of uplifting moments. It can help you communicate to others what you need to put forth your best effort.

You possess the power to welcome more fulfillment.

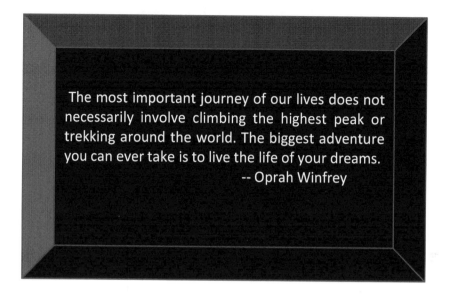

Advanced Self-Care

Life is full of unexpected events. We have the opportunity to view them as a chance to pause and rest. Sometimes interruptions let you know that you will burn out at your pace and in your current environment.

Whether your pause has a short or long duration, take advantage of this opportunity to embrace rest and rediscover yourself. Well rested, you will return strategic, stronger, and ready to pursue YOUR dream.

There are some famous people who have experienced setbacks. Some onlookers believed they could not achieve the same support they had prior to their challenge. They were shamed in the public media. But, during their rest, they formed new alliances, uncovered better- fit mentors, developed a bigger vision, and proceeded with fortitude.

> "When you stand and share your story in an empowering way, your story will heal you and your story will heal somebody else." -- Iyanla Vanzant

- After being arrested, DC's Mayor Marion Barry won re-election.
- After a well-publicized marital affair, Jay Z and Beyonce have become one of our nation's power couples.
- After being diagnosed with autism, Tom Stoltman became the strongest man in the world.
- After being diagnosed with HIV, Magic Johnson became a business mogul.
- After embracing her vitiligo, Winnie Harlow became a world-famous model.
- After addressing years of depression and ADHD, Michael Phelps proceeded to win 23 Gold Olympic Medals.
- After surviving a cerebral aneurysm, I, Kellye Jones, have gone on to write two books.
- After surviving an abusive marriage, Tina Turner moved on to a new marriage and continued success.

Wheel of Life's Self-Care Assessment

Paul J. Meyer, the founder of the Success Motivation Institute, created the Wheel of Life to help his audience develop a more balanced life. He believed balance elevates attitude, and attitude undergirds satisfaction.

Imagine the center as your starting point toward satisfaction and the outer ring as maximized satisfaction.

Then shade each of the seven areas on the wheel up to your current level of satisfaction. Setting milestones toward your goal will elevate your endorphins (success hormones), confidence, problem-solving skills, and energy throughout your journey.

Your positive aura will attract potential collaborators. Your aura will also attract critics who may have a different value system, skill set, or vision, but you can determine the size of the role they will play in your goal. The insight from the Wheel of Life can be used in setting goals for self-care.

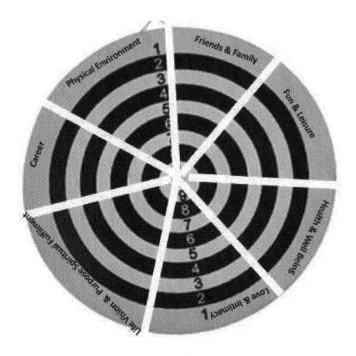

If your Wheel of Life has high markings in one category and low markings in another, do not rush to secure more success in the low-scoring category. Instead, maximize your areas with higher levels of success. It takes less energy to generate exponential advancements in an accomplished area than create awareness and success in a new area.

There is always room for collaboration or bartering when needed, in low-priority areas. Surpassing escalating milestones will extend your perceptions and elevate your expectations of success in other areas.

> I am not really good at being predictive, so I guess I'm willing to be surprised.
> Gwen Ifill

Good stress, or eustress, is the excitement and anticipation of what's next. It's the joy of waiting to open a surprise gift. The box or gift bag that stimulates your imagination.

Bad stress, or acute stress, is temporary but draining. It can positively or adversely impact your pain tolerance and temperance. The key is to understand its onset and develop coping or avoidance measures. Stretching your pain tolerance too far can push you beyond your pain threshold and into a state of chronic stress.

If unaddressed or misinterpreted, stress can have more severe side effects such as depression, adrenal gland cancer, congenital adrenal hyperplasia, Cushing's Syndrome, General Adaption Syndrome, and even suicide. The fight or flight hormone and muscle tightening occur when the body senses fear.

On the other hand, a deficiency in cortisol speeds up the aging process, can cause muscle pains, and reduce libido.

Maintain balance and uncover coping strategies for your best physical and social health.

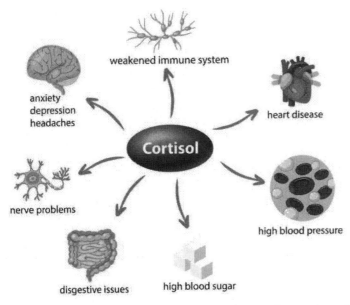

Timely peer affirmation may also reduce chronically high levels of the stress hormone cortisol.

Schedule a daily time for calls with peers or meals with a friend. Try to emulate times like the siesta and fiesta hours practiced in Spain. Unaddressed stress can cause neuroinflammation of the brain and spinal cord area.

"High stress affects the part of the brain responsible for judgment, memory, reasoning, and problem-solving."
-- Dr. Nadine Burke Harris

High stress is one of the internal causes of neuroinflammation in this frontal lobe. Micro stressors are repeated stressful events that can build a high-stress status if not addressed early. External trauma, such as a fall, car accident, or concussion can also cause neuroinflammation. The onset of post-concussion syndrome may not appear until three weeks after the injury. It is important to address headaches, stress, and injuries or they may disrupt sleep and tear down emotional reserves.

Insufficient self-care can lead to masking chronic physical conditions. Some health conditions, such as those listed below, are misdiagnosed as stress:

- Crohn's Disease
- Dysautonomia – breathing
- Episodic Ataxia – clumsiness
- Fibromyalgia
- Food allergies
- Food sensitivities
- Hypertension
- Lupus
- Stomach ulcers
- Thyroid disorders

Stay Agile. For example, YouTube started as a video dating site on February 14, 2005. After five days of not having one dating video uploaded, they converted it to a site for gathering all types of videos. A pivot is a change in strategy without a change in vision Eric Ries. Sometimes tweak, go left, or go right on your pathway to reach your ultimate goal. Retreating, rethinking, and repeating are not moving backward; it may be the move you need to make for superb grounding.

Setbacks are commas, not periods. Think of McDonald's success as a fast-food restaurant. Periodically, they will try a new menu item. In 1989, they introduced Mickey D's pizza. They did not have a presence in the pizza market. So, they sought to capture as many fast-food family dining customers as possible.

Well, there is one thing that custom pizza is not- fast. The complaints about the McPizza included a Pizza Hut ad calling it the McFrozen. The list of complaints led McDonald's to remove their Mickey D's pizza menu option. On the other hand, they are still innovating and doing well with their core product – the hamburger.

Chapter Sixteen:
Constructive and Motivational Feedback

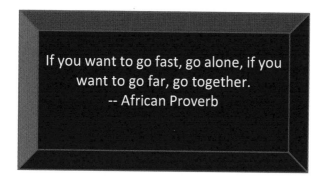

New opportunities are coming. Try to embrace a life full of commas and not just periods. Then you will attract supportive people who will listen and understand you.

Listeners and hearers are different. Listeners intentionally hear your words. Hearers generalize what they are hearing.

Create your team of listeners who will help you advance to your next level of success.

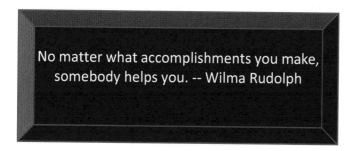

Below are some suggestions for mutual collaborations. Well-planned collaboration and constructive feedback support growth and empowerment.

Cheerleader- Someone to remind you of your great traits and ability to surpass your goals. Create a code to let them know when they need to call you back quickly. Make sure you reciprocate sincere encouragement. Everyone needs and enjoys uplifting.

Collaborator- Someone with whom you can share a list of what is needed and listen to their list of what is missing. Your collaborator will partner with you to complete the task, or you will help each other find resources.

Coach – Someone to remind you of your skills and resources for your most effective pathway to your solution. Establish a regular time for updates.

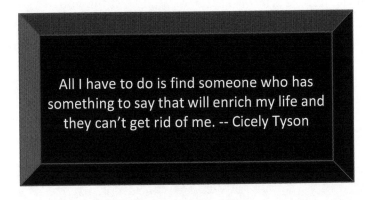

Keep going. The vision and pathway will become clear.

Fulfilled is defined as "satisfied or happy because of fully developing one's abilities or character. Being fulfilled is a process through failures and victories, rather than focusing on one specific moment."

Chapter Seventeen:
Making Your Next Move Forward

The Almost Millions of Dollars Mistake

Taking things one step further: if you uncover a specific project, cause, opportunity you are passionate about along your journey, find others with the same interests. Purpose promotes passion, vision, engagement, and fulfilment. Simply put – joy.

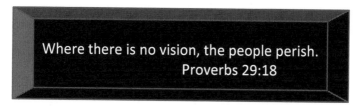

> Where there is no vision, the people perish.
> Proverbs 29:18

Mentor. Study Upward. Explore Outward.

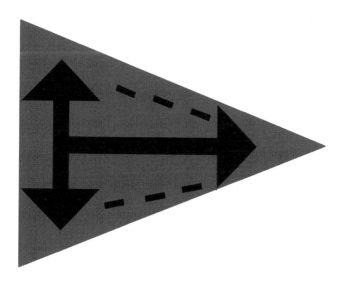

Establishing traction for a new concept requires communication with novices, experts, and peers. Seek diverse conversations while gathering insight, resources, and support.

Novices. They will ask and answer questions on what others may be missing. A little brother or sister may add to your vision. Sometimes they are not limited by all the things others say cannot be done. If you are looking to do something new or different with social media or computers, ask an adult, that does not use social media regularly, what features would help them use social media more.

Upward. Seek persons who are where you would like to be in five years. Research leaders in the local news and through Google. There are also organizations that can help you build a business model. Keep in mind, Asia Newson began her candle business at age 5.

Super Business Girl and **SCORE** are two examples of mentorship programs for entrepreneurs.

Outward. Asking friends for support with marketing. What looks and sounds appealing? Frequently updating your pulse on your audience for sustainability.

My mentor found a new artist he was looking to sponsor but wanted a second opinion. One day, he called me to his office and asked me to view some of the artist's work. He was looking to hire me as the manager of this artist's career.

After maybe five minutes of viewing the art, he asked, "Where do you envision seeing these historical figure profiles displayed?" I responded, "My mother is a fourth- grade teacher. I could envision her buying a stack of twenty to highlight famous American historical figures." He inquired, "At an elementary school?" Then proceeded to explain, "I am looking at the details in this picture. I envision hosting showings at museums and creating one-of-a-kind or limited-edition art pieces."

I responded, "I see school art at a purchase price of 4 for $20 and no individual sales."

Since our views were polarized, he asked me to host a focus group discussion to determine the art's value. I gathered 15 participants for the focus group. They were diverse in age, disposable income, love of art, and race, some were analytical introverts while others were talkative extroverts. The only thing I asked of all participants is that they provide honest feedback on the portraits.

We began the focus group with introductions and a light discussion about the participant's interest in art.

After everyone felt comfortable speaking in front of the group, I brought out the first piece of art.

The room was quiet. So, I brought out three additional works of art and displayed them side by side. When I asked, "Where do you envision seeing this art?" There were two responses.

1. In my grandmother's living room.
2. In a classroom.

When I asked, "How much would you pay for the art?" the responses varied between 3 for $20 and 5 for $20.

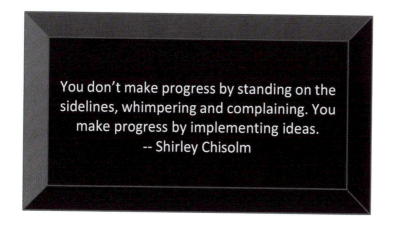

You don't make progress by standing on the sidelines, whimpering and complaining. You make progress by implementing ideas.
-- Shirley Chisolm

My mentor thanked me. He then stressed the importance of conducting focus groups whenever you are introducing a new idea. Do not assume others will support your idea. Even if he and I agreed on the same price, he would have still hosted a focus group.

Ultimately, it was better to walk with honesty, integrity, and purpose. Working with a reliable, diverse team allows you to move *FORWARD* in those areas.

> I knew well that the only way I could get that door open was to knock it down; because I knocked all of them down. -- Sadie Tanner Mossell Alexander

Successful Business Owners who stated their business before age 21

Name	Company/Service	Age (Years in Business)
Jack Bonneau	Jack's Stands & Marketplace	17 (8)
Tara Bosch	SmartSweets	22 (4)
Moziah Bridges	Mo's Bows	9 (12)
DJ Duarte	GreenWorx	8 (15)
Sanil Chawla	Hack+	23 (6)
Gabby Goodwin	GaBBY Bows	16 (9)
Neijae Graham-Henries	Barber	12 (4)
Jakhil Jackson	Project I Am (World Homelessness Awareness)	15 (4)
Christon "The Truth" Jones	$tocks 101, The Truth Success Series	11 (16)
Riya Karumanchi	SmartCane	19 (3)
Marsai Martin	Hollywood Executive Producer	19 (4)
Cory Nieves	Mr. Cory's Cookies	10 (4)
Kenan Pala	Kids4Community	19 (6)
Maya Penn	Maya's Ideas	23 (7)
Erin Smith	FacePrint	23 (7)
Michael Wren	Mikey's Munchies Vending	15 (4)

Successful Business Owners who stated their business after age 50

Name	Company/Service	Age Years in Business
Charles Flint	IBM	61 (112)
Leo Goodwin	GEICO	50 (87)
Steve Jobs	iPhone	50 (16)
Roy Kroc	McDonald's	52 (68)
Bernie Marcus	Home Depot	50 (45)
John Smith Pemberton	Coca Cola	55 (137)
Billy Porter	E Trade	54 (41)
Hartland Sanders	Kentucky Fried Chicken	65 (77)

Achieve It with HEART

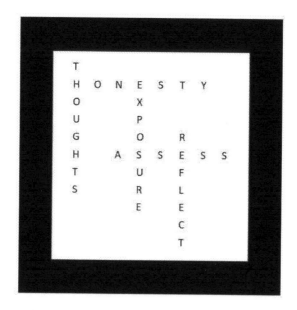

Move FORWARD toward your dream with regular HEART checks. I designed the real-time checklist below to double-check your resources, opportunities, and progress at milestones along your journey. Self-reflection is healthy, empowering, and engaging.

Most people are more ready to learn and remember more when they are engaged. They will push harder to obtain their goal because they feel good about the end result. Sometimes they will work so hard that they forget about self-care. It is important to remember to refuel your energy because you cannot give from an empty cup. Dr. David Rock of the NeuroLeadership Institute stated

Engagement is a state of being willing to do difficult things, to think deeply about issues, and develop new solutions. ... Interest, happiness, joy, and desire are **approach emotions**. This state is one of the increased dopamine levels, important for interest, and learning. The opposite is **withdrawal emotions** such as avoidance and anger.

> Each person deserves a day away in which no problems are confronted, no solutions searched for. Each of us needs to withdraw from the cares which will not withdraw from us. --Maya Angelou

HEART by Kellye Jones

Healthy Balance – Find your time commitment balance. Some people may choose to take evening breaks while others may choose to take off a day. Establish a time to enjoy other activities and hold yourself accountable so that you can return to your project refreshed.

How often do you currently take breaks from schoolwork or work?

_____
_____
_____
_____
_____

How often would you like to take breaks? Do you think you should have more quiet time or dedicate more time to perfecting a skill/ interest?

_____
_____
_____
_____
_____

Exposure and Expansion – Learn about different opportunities to apply your skills. Would you like to start a business, volunteer, learn a trade, invent a device, research rare diseases, or more? Ask people you know about your area of interest. Read articles and watch videos on your area of interest. Grow deeper in understanding.

After you answer these questions, make a list of who you will ask to mentor you.

_____
_____
_____
_____
_____

What one specific item about your plan would you like them to mentor? How to research, brand/ market, secure funding, select partners, and more. By selecting one area, you will help them understand their expected time commitment.

_____
_____
_____
_____
_____

> Thoughts have power, thoughts are energy. And you can make your world or break it by your own thinking. -- Susan Taylor

Assess – Develop a starting point and update a system to measure your progress. Some possible areas to research, are brand/ market, secure funding, select partners, and more. Then create a timeline and platform for tracking your progress. You can write, video record, photograph, collage, and more your progress.

What are your first three goals? How will you track your progress?

- _____
- _____
- _____

Reflect- Scale it.

List the items you do in your free time weekly. Then reflect on how they can help you move closer to your goal or distract you from your goal. Write an H next to the helpers and D next to the distractors. Is there one distractor you can spend less time doing for thirty days? Over the 30 days, list the things you are doing, during the additional free time, to help you get closer to your goal.

_____
_____
_____
_____
_____
_____

Thankfulness – Give and accept accolades. Affirmations remind us that we are on the right track. Who did you send a thank you letter to over the last thirty days? Who will you send a thank you card to next week?

_____
_____
_____
_____
_____
_____

> Life is like an egg: you have to be patient and careful with it or it will break.
> -- Langston Hughes

Chapter Eighteen:
Get it!

People have more than cookie-cutter challenges, requiring more than cookie-cutter hearers and solutions. We need active listeners and more options.

In the picture below, Mihaly Csikszentmihalyi's Flow State provides insight into the role of a life coach and a licensed clinical therapist or counselor. The goal is to stay within the FLOW area to more effectively and peacefully reach your vision.

Sometimes life's challenges may cause a person to drift into a situational/ temporary state of anxiety. During such times, a person may feel like they do not have the skills to complete a challenge. Or the person may believe they have the skills but may be uncertain about the best pathway to use their skills most effectively.

Temporary anxiety is when the challenge is mundane and the person is overly qualified. The question then becomes, "How do I stay engaged to avoid errors?" or "What are some of the underutilized talents that I can use to enjoy a side business or incorporate into volunteering?

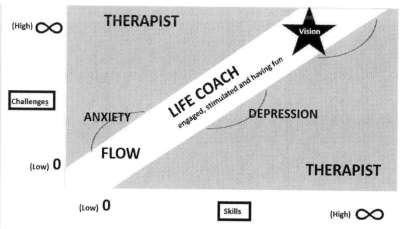

It can be tough trying to uncover your best pathways to greater achievement on your own. If it were easy, you would have already done it. If your friends had the answer, you would have already accomplished it. Staying in your FLOW zone and striving towards your goal takes an authentic look at your character strengths and a continued belief as well as a clear vision of your end goal. Using only half of your strengths or working super hard will leave you with halfway results.

It's time to prioritize your interest and excitement. It's time for that big smile that says, "I got this."

It's time for you to walk in YOUR FLOW.

In both scenarios, there are lulls that can be overcome with the assistance of a life coach.

Life coaches help people uncover their strengths. They work with clients who are closer to the FLOW State.

A life coach can help you:
- Navigate beyond uniform responses
- Highlight underutilized character strengths
- Unveil naturally creative skills
- Innovate new pathways to sustainable solutions
- Uncover collaborative opportunities
- Utilize objective benchmarks
- Navigate beyond uniform responses
- Tackle complex issues

People who have a prolonged state of anxiety may choose to work with a psychologist or psychiatrist.

Utilize the Ready to Go Litmus Test with peers to measure your growth in conveying details.

Explain your new concept for innovation or duplication to multiple peers with different interests. You are checking to see if there are any additional questions you need to answer about the process and outcome. You are seeking understanding not their approval of your idea. Ask them how you performed on the attached questionnaire.

Best of luck! Have fun and go for it!

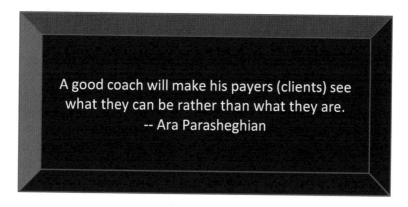

> A good coach will make his payers (clients) see what they can be rather than what they are.
> -- Ara Parasheghian

Litmus Test by Kellye Jones

Based on the knowledge I have today....						
	Strongly Agree	Agree	Neutral	Strongly Agree	Disagree	Strongly Disagree
1. I can describe my target audience.						
2. I can describe my strengths.						
3. I have eclectic filters and they address my audience/ team.						
4. I have established milestones.						
5. I understand the uniqueness of my vision.						
6. I have benchmarks for success.						
7. I can describe success.						
8. I have identified teammates.						
9. I have identified motivators.						
10. I have identified my need to take a break indicator(s).						

> You don't make progress by standing on the sidelines, whimpering and complaining. You make progress by implementing ideas. -- Shirley Chisholm

You will often hear presenters say, "Know your audience." I agree it is crucial to know the interests of your audience, but audiences change. On the other hand, your uniqueness and character strengths are with you everywhere you go.

Master your understanding of your strengths' versatility, and your excellence will shine in every setting.

Chapter Nineteen
Pay it Forward

Embarking on a new goal should be fun. What could be more fun than developing your talents, and strengths, and leading your team to reach a fulfilling goal? Stay ready for new opportunities to learn even in the most unexpected places.

It will be one of the most rewarding leaps you will ever make. You will be amazed by all the internal and external resources you have at your fingertips to make a difference for yourself and others. Your enthusiasm and awareness will draw like-minded persons to collaborate with you in your venture.

As you begin to walk in your vision, remember three things.
1. Develop a mentee. They will ask you the questions that will make you a keener leader. They will have fewer traditional filters and limitations. Your mentee will ask, "Why?" and keep your brand innovative.
2. Master Volunteering. During the tough days when it seems like a lot is going wrong, you can reflect on that time of giving to complete strangers and know you are making a difference.
3. Allocate "me time." Block out time to develop and define your strengths, talents, and challenges. This will ensure a pathway of success that best compliments you. It will lead to the greatest fulfillment in whatever you do.

Wouldn't you love to have more passion and clarity about your purpose? Would you love to walk in it knowing that the difference you are making is more than temporary?

We live in an interdependent world. Learn, teach, and grow in this world.

One morning, I picked up my director, at a local hotel, for a day of sales calls. We ate breakfast at the buffet while planning our day of sales calls.

As we were leaving, I asked him to give me a few minutes to return to the buffet and grab a few bananas. He preponderantly looked at me and said, "OK." Maybe he was thinking, "Since it is customary for directors to treat their salesmen to lunch during sales calls, why is she taking additional food?"

Less than five miles away from the hotel, I stopped at a red light, proceeded to roll my window down and hand the bananas to a homeless man. My manager said, "Wow! I stay at hotels all the time, and I never thought to take a banana for the homeless persons I would pass during the day.

Where did you get that idea?"

I explained, "My dad and I spent many weekends in Manhattan. The first couple of times, we passed a homeless person, I asked my dad to give them money. Instead, he would stop by a local grocery store and buy pieces of fruit. I would then go back and give the person the fruit in a bag and watch their face as they opened it. Some would say 'Thank you' or 'God bless you.' Others would throw it in the trash. The smiles on the faces of those who said thank you always overshadowed the tosses in the trash." My director replied, "Thank you. You taught me something new."

About The Author

Empaths see a need and pour 150% of themselves into helping others, which often leads to them ignoring their own critical signs of emotional and physical fatigue. They can become increasingly engaged in supporting others until the thin line between pain tolerance and pain threshold becomes blurred.

One night, while preparing a lesson for my students, the words before me became blurred. I used three sources to frame my bible study lessons- the bible, the Strongs Concordance, and the Parallel Bible. I would also use periodic breaks to work on my school lessons referencing high school workbooks, high school text books, the computer, and handwritten notes for contemporary context. As I shifted reading the three sources, the words became harder to decipher. After 15 minutes of trying to dismiss my reading challenges, I closed my books and went to bed.

When I woke up, things were different. I was not sure if my daily far-reaching tasks, sluggishness, or something else was not right. Hours later, I scheduled a next-day appointment with my doctor. That evening, trusting the mind over matter, I began preparing for my lesson again.

My vision was worse, and my attempt to read lasted less than five minutes. I would not give up; so, I kept taking small breaks with my eyes closed and then continued to read. Suddenly, a sharp pain traveled from my temple to the back of my head. The pain felt like the tip of a safety pin was scraping my head. The intensity was unlike anything I had ever experienced.

I prayed my students would forgive me for resting.

I did not believe in quitting. I turned off the lights and closed my eyes. As I tried to relax, thoughts of letting down my students kept nagging me. How could I get so sick that I could not prepare for my lesson? My only response was, "I should have started working on my assignment earlier." I scheduled a doctor's appointment immediately hoping he would provide a solution that would allow my vision to get better. I wanted to finish my lesson in time for class.

My son and daughter were in my class. Teaching the class allowed us to talk about my lessons for days after the class and find the moral of the lesson in daily activities. Sometimes I would hear my daughter teaching her friends one of my previous lessons. When I told her I was not feeling well and I might not be able to teach the class, she brought me an aspirin and told me to rest. She said, "Mommy you have to teach our class. Take a nap and you will feel better soon." I tried but my head hurt so much that I just could not sleep.

That afternoon, I went to the doctor's office. It was one of the longest waits I believe I have ever experienced in a doctor's office. The anticipation of an answer, hope, caused me to arrive at my doctor's office 30 minutes early. I remember sitting there thinking about my daughter's belief that I would be good to go in no time. At the same time, I could not get beyond my blurred vision to read and complete the sign-in information. Eventually, I sat down and began to comb through magazines looking for stylish glasses. Maybe glasses were the solution.

"Kellye Jones, the doctor, will see you now," said the nurse. Finally, some answers, or so I thought. After explaining my symptoms and family history, the doctor suggested an eye exam, sleeping pills, and almost every non-prescribed painkiller under the kitchen sink. Each time she suggested a treatment plan, I requested a CT scan. After her sixth suggestion, I asked a sixth time for a CT scan. I was relentless.

Finally, based on the fact that I was not willing to give in, and listed
- My maternal grandfather died of a cerebral aneurysm
- My maternal uncle died of a cerebral aneurysm
- My maternal aunt died of and cerebral aneurysm
- My paternal uncle died of an aortic aneurysm

She told me to reduce my stress. She gave me a prescription for headaches, an ophthalmologist referral, and ordered my CT scan. She said she was impressed with my knowledge my family history. She still did not believe I had an aneurysm. She thought I was too composed to be in the type of pain I was describing. Sometimes a person's pain tolerance can be mistaken for not exceeding their pain threshold. This is why aneurysms have a high rate of mortality.

While waiting for the CT scan, I had a doctor's visit with the ophthalmologist. He prescribed glasses but he felt as though my headaches and vision challenges were stress related. He said the stiffness in my neck and challenges should be checked by a neurologist. Neurologists work with patients who have aneurysms.

Within a week, I found out that I had an aneurysm. I spent the next six Fridays having MRIs or waiting in the ER with overnight hospital admission for my headaches. During my sixth Friday visit, I overheard my physician say, "We are waiting for it to burst to perform surgery." Keep in mind, according to the Brain Aneurysm Foundation, 50% of ruptures are fatal, and 66% of patients who have ruptures suffer permanent neurological damage.

My daughter prayed and fasted for the best doctor. Immediately, I began searching for other physicians, even in other states. I was looking for the best neurosurgeon available. I found the top four neurosurgeons in the United States. My parents were going to fly me to Barrow Neurological Institute in Phoenix, Az. Then a colleague recommended Dr. Rosenwasser at Jefferson Hospital in Philadelphia. Dr. Rosenwasser was within driving distance, and I loved the fact that I could travel to his office with my family.

Dr. Robert H. Rosenwasser viewed my MRI with contrast results the following Tuesday at 4 pm and scheduled an appointment for 7 am the next morning, in Philadelphia. We drove seven hours from North Carolina to Jefferson University Hospital in Philadelphia that night. After meeting with Dr. Rosenwasser, he walked outside the room, and told the nurse, "Her aneurysm could rupture at any moment. Admit her."

When I arrived in my hospital room, I prayed for these three things.

First, I thanked God for healing me. I just believed with all my heart healing was on the way. I believed God had more in store for me to do. A few years prior, I applied for admission to the Duke Divinity School. The admission counselor told me about her vision for me. Funny how uplifting conversations can give you hope in the most difficult times. Instead of fear, I felt full of victory and purpose.

Two, I asked God to reveal my stressors and opportunities to reduce stress so that I could lead a healthier life. I grew up in an affirming family environment with lots of laughter. Later on, I became the brunt of many jokes. I laughed because I loved to laugh. But truthfully, I was hurting inside. As I began to reflect on the source of my laughter and the loss of my authentic self, I asked for relief from the constant ridicule or a way to cope during the process.

I quickly learned that one size fits all self-care had not worked for me. I knew that I missed the big city lights of New York City and the spectacular lights of Disney World. So, I hired an electrician to build a unique rope lighting design in our basement. I would sit in the basement with my children watching the beautiful lights and fish in our fish tank while they watched TV. That was peace.

Three, I knew HIS saving grace, the victory from missed diagnosis and misdiagnosis, was for a greater purpose and ministry. So, I asked HIM to show me my daily and long-term goals in disrupting overly generalized diagnoses, misdiagnoses, and missed diagnoses. I am blessed to be here to say I am a survivor. I have a purpose.

Someone's quality of life is being made better because you dreamed, cared for, and committed to making a difference. Life is getting better because you are walking into your best self.

Thank you in advance for your kindness and readiness to walk boldly in your purpose.

Kellye Jones is a divorced mother of three children. She is a Certified Life Coach, who holds a Communications degree from the University of North Carolina at Chapel Hill and is currently pursuing an M.Ed. at Liberty University. She has also received two TEACCH for Autism Certificates and a Cognitive Behavioral Therapy. Once a month, she (Coach KJ) and Dr. Valentina co-host the Moving Forward Podcast Stories of Triumph. The link to many of their previous podcast can be found at https://forwardlifecoach.com/moving-forward-podcast The Former NCAA Student-Athletes Stories of Triumph YouTube Series, which includes an interview with Cornell Brown of the Baltimore Ravens **Super Bowl XXXV** Championship Team, George Koonce of the **Super Bowl XXXI Team**, NFL Football Player Reggie Clark, and NBA Basketball Players John Wallace and Jeff McInnis as well as many other dominant NCAA student athletes who are now successful coaches and trainers can also be found at https://forwardlifecoach.com.

In 2023, Coach KJ and Dr. Felecia Harris will begin cohosting the podcast "Solutions" to provide listeners with more pathways to address neurological and immunological challenges.

Coach KJ can be reached at TheKellyeJones@gmail.com
Dr. Valentina can be reached at drvalentinapsyd@gmail.com

> People don't always have the vision, and the secret for the person with the vision is to stand up. It takes a lot of courage. -- Natalie Cole

Glossary

(Definitions from the Merriam Webster Dictionary)

Alexithymia - inability to identify and express or describe one's feelings

Altruism - unselfish regard for or devotion to the welfare of others

Ambivert - a person having characteristics of both extrovert and introvert

Aneurysm - an abnormal blood-filled bulge of a blood vessel and especially an artery resulting from weakening (as from disease) of the vessel wall

Anhedonia - a psychological condition characterized by inability to experience pleasure in normally pleasurable acts

Assimilation - the process of receiving new facts or of responding to new situations in conformity with what is already available to consciousness

Asymptomatic - not causing, marked by, or presenting with signs or symptoms of infection, illness, or disease

Baseline – a known measure or position used) to calculate or locate something

Bipolar - having or marked by two mutually repellent forces or diametrically opposed natures or views

Body Language - the gestures, movements, and mannerisms by which a person or animal communicates with others

Catalyst - an agent that provokes or speeds significant change or action

Claustrophobia - abnormal dread of being in closed or narrow spaces

Collaborate - to work jointly with others or together especially in an intellectual endeavor

Compliments - an expression of esteem, respect, affection, or admiration

Constructive - promoting improvement or development

Contextual Reference - the <u>interrelated</u> conditions in which something exists or occurs

Cookie-cutter - marked by lack of originality or distinction

Cortisol - a glucocorticoid $C_{21}H_{30}O_5$ produced by the adrenal <u>cortex</u> upon stimulation by ACTH that mediates various metabolic processes (such as gluconeogenesis), has anti-inflammatory and immunosuppressive properties, and whose levels in the blood may become elevated in response to physical or psychological stress

Deconstructing – the process of to taking apart or examine (something) in order to reveal the basis or composition often with the intention of exposing biases, flaws, or inconsistencies

Depression - a state of feeling sad

Diplomatic - employing <u>tact</u> and conciliation especially in situations of stress

Discernment - the quality of being able to <u>grasp</u> and comprehend what is <u>obscure</u>

Dopamine - a monoamine $C_8H_{11}NO_2$ that is a decarboxylated form of dopa and that occurs especially as a neurotransmitter in the brain

Downtime - inactive time (such as time between periods of work)

Dual Personality Disorder - a <u>personality disorder</u> that is characterized by the presence of two or more distinct and complex identities or personality states each of which becomes dominant and controls behavior from time to time to the exclusion of the others and results from disruption in the integrated functions of consciousness, memory, and identity

Dysarthria - difficulty in articulating words due to disease of the central nervous system

Embarking - to make a start

Emotionally - markedly aroused or agitated in feeling or sensibilities

Empath - one who experiences the emotions of others: a person who has empathy for others

Endorphins - any of a group of endogenous peptides (such as enkephalin) found especially in the brain that bind chiefly to opiate receptors and produce some pharmacological effects (such as pain relief) like those of opiates

Engage - to hold the attention of

Euphoric - marked by a feeling of great happiness and excitement

Eustress - a positive form of stress having a beneficial effect on health, motivation, performance, and emotional well-being such as a promotion or vacation, feel-good chemicals called endorphins are released

Extrovert - a typically gregarious and unreserved person who enjoys and seeks out social interaction

Fortitude - strength of mind that enables a person to encounter danger or bear pain or adversity with courage

Hare Krishna - a member of a religious group dedicated to the worship of the Hindu god Krishna

Homesick - longing for home and family while absent from them

Imbibing - to receive into the mind and retain

Imposter Syndrome - a psychological condition that is characterized by persistent doubt concerning one's abilities or accomplishments accompanied by the fear of being exposed as a fraud despite evidence of one's ongoing success

Intentionality - done by intention or design

Intrinsic - originating or due to causes within a body, organ, or part

Introvert - a typically reserved or quiet person who tends to be introspective and enjoys spending time alone

Like-minded - having a like disposition or purpose: of the same mind or habit of thought

Misophonia - a condition in which one or more common sounds (such as the ticking of a clock, the hum of a fluorescent light, or the chewing or breathing of another person) cause an atypical emotional response (such as disgust, distress, panic, or anger) in the affected person hearing the sound

Neurologically – a branch of medicine concerned especially with the structure, function, and diseases of the nervous system

Nimbleness - marked by quick, alert, clever conception, comprehension, or resourcefulness

Novice - a person admitted to probationary membership in a religious community

Optimal - most desirable or satisfactory

Overgeneralized - to make excessively vague or general statements about something or someone

Paradigm shift - an important change that happens when the usual way of thinking about or doing something is replaced by a new and different way

Phobias - an exaggerated usually inexplicable and illogical fear of a particular object, class of objects, or situation

Pivot - a usually marked change an adjustment or modification made (as to a product, service, or strategy) in order to adapt or improve

Reciprocate - to give and take mutually

Resilient - tending to recover from or adjust easily to misfortune or change

Respite - an interval of rest or relief

Self-Affirmation - the act of affirming one's own worthiness and value as an individual for beneficial effect (such as increasing one's confidence or raising self-esteem)

Self- Assessment - the act or process of analyzing and evaluating oneself or one's actions

Self-Awareness - an awareness of one's own personality or individuality

Self-efficacy – an awareness of one's own power to produce an effect
Self-esteem - a confidence and satisfaction in oneself
Self-preservation - preservation of oneself from destruction or harm
Self-worth – a sense of one's own value as a human being
Tangible - capable of being precisely identified or realized by the mind
Tedious - tiresome because of length or dullness : BORING
Tone - accent or inflection expressive of a mood or emotion
Underutilized - not fully utilized
Unmask - to reveal the true nature of : EXPOSE

References

8 dimensions of well-being. Colorado State University Pueblo. (n.d.). https://www.csupueblo.edu/health-education-and-prevention/8-dimension-of-well-being.html

Active-duty military find PTSD relief through individual cognitive therapy. Duke Health Referring Physicians. (2017, January 31). https://physicians.dukehealth.org/articles/active-duty-military-find-ptsd-relief-through-individual-cognitive-therapy

Admin. (2018, September 2). *Synergy and dysergy*. Indiaclass. https://indiaclass.com/synergy-and-dysergy/

Agarwal, N., Thakkar, R., & Than, K. (n.d.). *Sports-related Head Injury*. AANS. https://www.aans.org/Patients/Neurosurgical-Conditions-and-Treatments/Sports-related-Head-Injury#

Alber, R. (2013, March 4). How are happiness and learning connected? Edutopia. Retrieved March 28, 2023, from https://www.edutopia.org/blog/happiness- learning-connection-rebecca-alber

Asghar, N., Ali, M., Hannah, T., Li, A. Y., Asfaw, Z., Hrabarchuk, E. I., Quinones, A., McCarthy, L., Vasan, V., Murtaza-Ali, M., Lin, A., Alasadi, H., Nakadar, Z., Schupper, A. J., Gometz, A., Lovell, M. R., & Choudhri, T. F. (2023, August 23). *Concussion Incidence and Recovery of Neurocognitive Dysfunction Among Youth Athletes Taking Antibiotics: A Preliminary, Multicenter Retrospective Cohort Study*. Human Kinetics. https://journals.humankinetics.com/view/journals/ijatt/aop/article-10.1123-ijatt.2022-0111/article-10.1123-ijatt.2022-0111.xml

Authentic strengths advantage. (n.d.). Retrieved March 28, 2023, from https://authenticstrengths.com/wp-content/uploads/2020/05/ASA- Microlearning-Course-Library-May-2020- v12.pdf

Baby, D. P., & Valllie, S. (2022, November 14). *Pragmatic language disorder (social communication disorder)*. WebMD. https://www.webmd.com/children/what-is-pragmatic-language-disorder

Bales, R. (2023, July 31). *Xerox Alto: Everything You Need To Know*. History. https://history-computer.com/xerox-alto-guide/

Barehem, H. (2023, March 16). College graduation statistics. Yahoo! Finance. Retrieved March 27, 2023, from https://finance.yahoo.com/news/college- graduation-statistics-035013402.html

Barker, A. (2016, September 24). *5 habits to a fulfilled life*. HuffPost. Retrieved March 28, 2023, from https://www.huffpost.com/entry/5-habits-to- a-fulfilled-l_b_8188458#

Bethea, A. (2019, August 16). *Marsai Martin is just one of 15 young black entrepreneurs making bank*. BET. Retrieved April 29, 2023, from https://www.bet.com/article/zjw3eo/marsai-martin-and- more-young-black-entrepreneurs-making-bank

The Big Five Personality Test. Open-Source Psychometrics Project. (n.d.). Retrieved March 28, 2023, from https://openpsychometrics.org/tests/IPIP- BFFM/

Biography.com Editors. (n.d.). *Michael Phelps Biography*. Biography.com. https://www.biography.com/athlete/michael-phelps

Bradberry, T. (2022, October 12). *9 signs that you're an Ambivert*. Forbes. Retrieved March 27, 2023, from https://www.forbes.com/sites/travisbradberry/2016/04/26/9-signs-that-youre-an-ambivert/?sh=2c5b2123145b

Byrne, J. (2021a, October 7). *How does a psychiatrist make a diagnosis so quickly?*. Cognitive Psychiatry of Chapel Hill. https://www.cognitive-psychiatry.com/how-does-a-psychiatrist-make-a-diagnosis-so-quickly/

Brown, J. (2022, July 21). *Black business owners under the age of 20 on critical early success lessons*. CNBC. Retrieved April 29, 2023, from https://www.cnbc.com/2022/06/19/black-business-owners-under-the-age-of-20-on-early-success-lessons.html

Can a mental health diagnosis be removed? Immrama Institute. (2022, September 21). Retrieved March 28, 2023, from https://immramainstitute.com/sleeping/can-a- mental-health-diagnosis-be-removed

Can PTSD be mistaken for ADHD?. PTSD UK |. (n.d.). https://www.ptsduk.org/can-ptsd-be-mistaken-for-adhd/?fbclid=IwAR0zNArW2KaPg59i69d4MCX2bbTr28642nZDqTyKrifEn7nCJOFWP9oNwZs_aem_AU0SXkPiov6xMe_DTuhU8t6URXL9nKc2lnQ1oFysI-YoctxsJL1MeoB5SdbP0SO5-cQ&mibextid=Zxz2cZ

Can childhood PTSD be mistaken for autism?. PTSD UK |. (n.d.-a). https://www.ptsduk.org/can-childhood-ptsd-be-mistaken-for-autism/?fbclid=IwAR3gqLkTjMdoDjmuhQDcDgkQZr4xsGbFnhazU8Ai45r7WCerId11IYwFdCk_aem_AU3dKBUB6VP2dyc6_Sp7LK6TCPjoNfUETvvhn3ffxeO3qenl3o5hzAmDb8AhvK2WGjw&mibextid=Zxz2cZ

Ceschi, A., Sartori, R., & Dickert, S. (2016). Grit or honesty- humility? new insights into the moderating role of personality between the health impairment process and counterproductive work behavior. *Frontiers in Psychology,* 7. https://doi.org/10.3389/fpsyg.2016.01799

Chamberlain, L. (2023, April 24). *Strongman Tom Stoltman reveals how going to the gym ... - men's health.* Strongman Tom Stoltman Reveals How Going to the Gym Changed His Opinion on Autism. https://www.menshealth.com/uk/health/a43683392/tom-stoltman-on-autism-diagnosis/

Chris, F. (2010). How the opinion of others affects our valuation of objects. Frontiers in Computational Neuroscience, 4. https://doi.org/10.3389/conf.fnins.2010.01.00 001

Cleary, E. (2022, November 16). *Learning styles: The vark model.* simpleshow. Retrieved March 28, 2023, from https://simpleshow.com/blog/learning-styles- the-vark-model/

Dutton, J. (2021, July 28). *How swimming saved Michael Phelps: An ADHD story.* ADDitude. https://www.additudemag.com/michael-phelps-adhd-advice-from-the-olympians-mom/

EB O'Donnell MB;Cascio CN;Tinney F;Kang Y;Lieberman MD;Taylor SE;An L;Resnicow K;Strecher VJ;, F. (2015, February 17). Self- affirmation alters the brain's response to health messages and subsequent behavior change. Proceedings of the National Academy of Sciences of the United States of America. Retrieved March 27, 2023, from https://pubmed.ncbi.nlm.nih.gov/25646442/

Elaine Houston, B. S. (2022, November 18). *12 strength-based skills & activities to boost your practice.* PositivePsychology.com. Retrieved March 28, 2023, from https://positivepsychology.com/strength- based-skills-activities/

Elias, M. (2022, November 23). *51 autism statistics: How many people have autism?.* Discovery ABA - At-Home ABA Therapy. https://www.discoveryaba.com/statistics/how-many-people-have-autism#:

☐ empathy test - determine your level of empathy for free. ☐ Empathy Test - Determine Your Level of Empathy for Free. (n.d.). Retrieved March 28, 2023, from https://psycho-tests.com/test/empathy-test

Evans, K. D. (2017, January 19). *Asia Newson has a business that's literally lit.* Andscape. Retrieved April 29, 2023, from https://andscape.com/features/asia-newson-super-business-girl/

Examining the hierarchical influences of the big-five dimensions and anxiety sensitivity on anxiety symptoms in children. *Frontiers in Psychology, 10.* https://doi.org/10.3389/fpsyg.2019.01185

Faria, J. (2023a, August 29). *U.S. retailers by ad spend 2022.* Statista. https://www.statista.com/statistics/261956/ad-spend-of-selected-retailers-in-the-us/

Faria, J. (2023b, September 6). *Burger King: Ad spend in the U.S. 2022.* Statista. https://www.statista.com/statistics/306694/ad-spend-burger-king-usa/

Feldman, J. (2022, October 12). How to pass a *pre-employment personality test.* TopResume. Retrieved March 27, 2023, from https://www.topresume.com/career- advice/how-to-pass-the-pre-employment- personality- test

Ghlionn, J. M. (2023, April 24). *Doctor who helped broaden autism spectrum "very sorry" for over-diagnosis.* New York Post. https://nypost.com/2023/04/24/doctor-who-broadened-autism-spectrum-sorry-for-over-diagnosis/

Ghosh, U. (2016, March 31). Don't feel like an extrovert or introvert? 7 signs you are an ambivert. Hindustan Times. Retrieved March 28, 2023, from https://www.hindustantimes.com/health-and- fitness/don-t-feel-like-an-extrovert-or- introvert-7-signs- you-are-an-ambivert/story- HWrru2VljH3s3AyBFCKDhJ.html

Goewey, D. J. (2017, December 7). 85 percent of what we worry about never happens.

Harris, N. B. (2014, September 11). *How childhood trauma affects health across a lifetime.* Nadine Burke Harris: How childhood trauma affects health across a lifetime | TED Talk. https://www.ted.com/talks/nadine_burke_harris_how_childhood_trauma_affects_health_across_a_lifetime

Helgoe, D. L. (2014, April 7). 3 unexpected signs that you're an introvert. Oprah.com. Retrieved March 27, 2023, from https://www.oprah.com/inspiration/signs- youre-secretly-an-introvert

Henderson, R. by E. (2022, March 24). *Study shows prevalence and misdiagnosis of post-concussive syndrome in children after mild head injury.* News. https://www.news-medical.net/news/20220324/Study-shows-prevalence-and-misdiagnosis-of-post-concussive-syndrome-in-children-after-mild-head-injury.aspx

Hendler, N. (2016). Why Chronic Pain Patients are Misdiagnosed 40 to 80% of the Time? Research Gate-Journal on Recent Advances in Pain , 94–98.https://doi.org/DOI:10.5005/jp-journals- 10046-0051

Hollander, A. (2023, June 29). *70+ Autism Statistics, Facts & Demographics*. At-Home ABA Therapy. https://www.bridgecareaba.com/blog/autism-statistics

Home Page. SCORE. (n.d.). Retrieved March 28, 2023, from https://www.score.org/

Horatio Alger Association. (2023, July 24). *News & announcements*. Horatio Alger. https://horatioalger.org/members/detail/david-l-steward/

House, C. (2001, September 1). *Inside the young mind*. endeavors. Retrieved March 27, 2023, from https://endeavors.unc.edu/fall2001/levine.htm

How Good Is Your Time Management? MindTools. (n.d.). Retrieved March 28, 2023, from https://www.mindtools.com/aavjrgg/how- good-is-your-time-management

How David Steward turned $2K from his father to a $14.5 billion business. The Forward Culture YouTube @theforwardculture. (2023, February 2). https://youtu.be/37XCCqjxl7s?si=bTuS9X8Q-Gg6McFw

HuffPost. Retrieved March 28, 2023, from https://www.huffpost.com/entry/85-of-what- we-worry-about_b_8028368

Hunter, L. (2017, February 2). *The 13-year-old entrepreneur changing the face of business in Detroit*. Forbes. Retrieved April 28, 2023, from https://www.forbes.com/sites/leahhunter/2017/01/10/the-13-year-old-entrepreneur-changing-the-face-of- business-in-detroit/?sh=3ef5b0ee1f1d

Jabali, M. (2023, June 2). *Black woman stuns doctors after awakening from catatonic state after 20 years*. Essence. https://www.essence.com/news/black-woman-medical-miracle-april-burrell/

Jones, K., & Pancheo-Cornejo, V. (2021, July 19). *Retired wrestler Sam seitles on moving forward with coach KJ and dr. Valentina*. BlogTalkRadio. https://www.blogtalkradio.com/braininjuryradio/2021/07/19/retired-wrestler-sam-seitles-on-moving-forward-with-coach-kj-and-dr-valentina

Jorge, R. E., & Arciniegas, D. B. (2014, March). *Mood disorders after TBI*. The Psychiatric clinics of North America. https://www.ncbi.nlm.nih.gov/pmc/articles/PMC3985339/

Kalish, D. (2011). Self-assessments. dougsguides. Retrieved March 27, 2023, from https://www.dougsguides.com/assesstop

Katharine Chan, Ms. (2022, July 26). *What are the top 5 most stressful life events?*. Verywell Mind. https://www.verywellmind.com/the-top-most-stressful-life-events-5547803

Kendra Cherry, Mse. (2023, March 14). *How mental health professionals use the DSM-5 Today*. Verywell Mind. https://www.verywellmind.com/the-diagnostic-and-statistical-manual-dsm-2795758#

Kerr, B. (2020, June 30). Depression among entrepreneurs is an epidemic nobody is talking about. The Hustle. Retrieved March 27, 2023, from https://thehustle.co/depression-among-entrepreneurs-is-an-epidemic-nobody-is-talking-about/

Khalid, S. (2023, July 13). *25 top-selling beers in America*. Yahoo! Finance. https://finance.yahoo.com/news/25-top-selling-beers-america-040529506.html

Kluger, J. (2018, February 15). *Why Amish people stay so healthy as they get older*. Time. https://time.com/5159857/amish-people-stay-healthy-in-old-age-heres-their-secret/

Lasarte, D. (2023, February 7). *Super Bowl LVII AD Watch: Less Crypto, more beer*. Quartz. https://qz.com/beer-ads-during-super-bowl-1850084498

Lehmann, J. A., & Seufert, T. (2017). The influence of background music on learning in the light of different theoretical perspectives and the role of working memory capacity. Frontiers in Psychology, 8. https://doi.org/10.3389/fpsyg.2017.01902

The Library of Congress. (n.d.). Retrieved March 27, 2023, from https://www.loc.gov/collections/edison- company-motion-pictures-and-sound- recordings/articles-and-essays/biography/life- of-thomas-alva-edison/

Life of Thomas Alva Edison: biography: articles and essays: inventing entertainment: The early motion pictures and sound recordings of the Edison Companies: digital collections: Library of Congress.

Linnstaedt, S. (2022, September 13). Chronic pain after trauma may depend on what stress gene variation you carry. The Conversation. Retrieved March 28, 2023, from https://theconversation.com/chronic-pain- after-trauma-may-depend-on-what-stress- gene-variation-you-carry-102021

Lyness, D. A. (Ed.). (2021, July). *Pandas and pans (for parents) - nemours kidshealth*. KidsHealth. Retrieved May 2, 2023, from https://kidshealth.org/en/parents/pandas.html

Mehta, K. (2022, October 12). *Older entrepreneurs outperform younger founders-shattering ageism*. Forbes. https://www.forbes.com/sites/kmehta/2022/08/23/older-entrepreneurs-outperform-younger-foundersshattering-ageism/?sh=bd45aa27a366

Matrin, D. S. (2021, April 16). *Mystery solved: Sudden onset of obsessive behaviors following infection - norton healthcare provider Louisville, KY.*. Norton Healthcare Provider. https://nortonhealthcareprovider.com/news/mystery-solved-sudden-onset-of-obsessive-behaviors-following-infection/

Mayo Foundation for Medical Education and Research. (2021, July 8). *Chronic stress puts your health at risk*. Mayo Clinic. Retrieved March 28, 2023, from https://www.mayoclinic.org/healthy- lifestyle/stress-management/in- depth/stress/art-20046037

McCain, A. (2023, June 28). *30 crucial customer service statistics to pay attention to [2023]: How businesses succeed*. Zippia. https://www.zippia.com/advice/customer-service-statistics/

Michele, Humes, C., Waller, J., & Lauren. (2022, December 24). *100% safe trypophobia test. this 2022 Quiz reveals your fear*. Quiz Expo. Retrieved March 28, 2023, from https://www.quizexpo.com/trypophobia-test/

Michele, Humes, C., Waller, J., & Lauren. (2022, December 24). *Claustrophobia test: Are you claustrophobic? 100% safe quiz*. Quiz Expo. Retrieved March 28, 2023, from https://www.quizexpo.com/claustrophobia- test/

Micromentor. MicroMentor. (n.d.). Retrieved March 28, 2023, from https://www.micromentor.org/mentors

Mills, P. by M. (2015, March 9). No you are not a visual/auditory/kinesthetic learner! Matter Of Facts. Retrieved March 28, 2023, from https://matteroffactsblog.wordpress.com/2015/03/09/no-you-are-not-a- visualauditorykinesthetic-learner/

New, J. (2015, January 27). College athletes greatly overestimate their chances of playing professionally. Retrieved March 27, 2023, from https://www.insidehighered.com/news/2015/01/27/college-athletes-greatly-overestimate- their-chances-playing-professionally

O'Brien, E. (2022, January 25). *The impact of ADHD on infection and the immune system*. Drug Topics. https://www.drugtopics.com/view/the-impact-of-adhd-on-infection-and-the-immune-system

Oliver, D. (2017, August 7). Study: Many Americans report feeling lonely, younger generations more so. US News. Retrieved March 29, 2023, from https://www.usnews.com/news/health-care-news/articles/2018-05-01/study-many- americans-report-feeling-lonely-younger- generations-more-so

PANDAS Network Healing Youth with PANS/AE. (2021, December 13). *Pandas symptoms checklistAH*. PANDAS Network. Retrieved May 2, 2023, from https://pandasnetwork.org/pandas-symptoms-checklist/

Parker, J. (2023, April 24). *Get the job you really want*. Zippia. https://www.zippia.com/answers/how-much-does-mcdonalds-spend-on-advertising/

Pedersen, T. (2023, May 10). *B12 and depression: What's the connection?* Psych Central. https://psychcentral.com/depression/b12-and-depression#

Planner Personality Quiz. Well Planned Gal. (2021, July 15). Retrieved March 28, 2023, from https://wellplannedgal.com/planner- personality/quiz/

Projectimplicit. Select a Test. (n.d.). Retrieved March 27, 2023, from https://implicit.harvard.edu/implicit/selectates t.html

Psycho-lexical approach. (2020). Encyclopedia of Personality and Individual Differences, 4145–4145. https://doi.org/10.1007/978-3-19-24612-3_302100

Raypole, C., & Gökbayrak, N. S. (2021, September 30). *PTSD and Bipolar Disorder: How They're Similar (and Different)*. Healthline. https://www.healthline.com/health/bipolar-disorder/ptsd-bipolar

Rollins, H. (n.d.). Are you an extrovert, introvert, or ambivert? THE MUSE. Retrieved March 27, 2023, from https://www.themuseatdreyfoos.com/top-stories/2018/02/21/are-you-an-extrovert- introvert-or-ambivert/

Roozitalab, S., Rahimzadeh, M., Mirmajidi, S. R., Ataee, M., & Esmaelzadeh Saeieh, S. (2021). *The relationship between infertility, stress, and quality of life with posttraumatic stress disorder in infertile women*. Journal of reproduction & infertility. https://www.ncbi.nlm.nih.gov/pmc/articles/PMC8669410/

Salsberry, M. (2023, August 22). *Critical Mechanics of Detractor recovery*. QuestionPro. https://www.questionpro.com/blog/mechanics-of-detractor-recovery/

Sensory quiz · sensory intelligence consulting. Sensory Intelligence Consulting. (2022, January 11). Retrieved March 28, 2023, from https://sensoryintelligence.com/sensory-quiz/

Singh, R., Turner, R. C., Nguyen, L., Motwani, K., Swatek, M., & Lucke-Wold, B. P. (2016). *Pediatric traumatic brain injury and autism: Elucidating shared mechanisms.* Behavioural neurology. https://www.ncbi.nlm.nih.gov/pmc/articles/PMC5198096/

Staff, E. (2019, August 20). *Meet 16 teen founders who are building big businesses -- and making big money.* Entrepreneur. Retrieved April 29, 2023, from https://www.entrepreneur.com/leadership/meet-16-teen-founders-who-are-building-big-businesses/337852

staff, H. (2022, September 25). *A guide to the differences and similarities of autism and CPTSD.* https://healthmatch.io/ptsd/cptsd-and-autism#what-is-ptsd

Stoewen, D. L. (2017, August). *Dimensions of Wellness: Change Your Habits, change your life.* The Canadian veterinary journal = La revue veterinaire canadienne. https://www.ncbi.nlm.nih.gov/pmc/articles/PMC5508938Person.

(2011, May 25). *the Oprah Winfrey Show finale.* Oprah.com. Retrieved March 28, 2023, from https://www.oprah.com/oprahshow/the- oprah-winfrey-show- finale_1/all#ixzz6bmypkgqs

Survey: 1 in 10 physicians admit to having Suicidal thoughts. Kaiser Health News. (2023, March 8). Retrieved March 27, 2023, from https://khn.org/morning- breakout/survey-1-in-10-physicians-admit-to- having-suicidal-thoughts/

Sussex Publishers. (n.d.). *Hexaco.* Psychology Today. Retrieved March 28, 2023, from https://www.psychologytoday.com/us/basics/ hexaco

Taylor, D. (2020, September 5). The incredible true story of Disney's Oswald the Lucky Rabbit. Collider. Retrieved March 28, 2023 from https://collider.com/disney-oswald- the-lucky-rabbit-history-explained/

Taylor, J. (2019, August 5). *Perception is not reality.* Psychology Today. Retrieved March 28, 2023, from https://www.psychologytoday.com/us/blog/th e-power-prime/201908/perception-is-not- reality

Team, M. (2023, February 18). *Depth psychology: History and meaning.* Meridian University. https://meridianuniversity.edu/content/depth-psychology-history-and-meaning#

Team, T. U. (2023, June 15). *How Michael Phelps' ADHD helped him make olympic history.* Understood. https://www.understood.org/en/articles/celebrity-spotlight-how-michael-phelps-adhd-helped-him-make-olympic-history

Thompson, D. (2023, February 23). Almost two- thirds of U.S. doctors, nurses feel burnt out at work: Poll. US News. Retrieved March 27, 2023, from https://www.usnews.com/news/health-news/articles/2023-02-23/almost-two-thirds- of-u-s-doctors-nurses-feel-burnt-out-at-work- poll

Thor, E. (2022, February 11). Big five test: Personalitopia: Erik Thor. Personalitopia. Retrieved March 27, 2023, from https://www.personalitopia.com/big-five-test/

Together. Retrieved March 27, 2023, from https://www.physicianleaders.org/

True, G. (2022, March 30). *Autism and Pans Pandas & Handout.* Aspire. Retrieved May 2, 2023, from https://aspire.care/families-parents-caregivers/autism-and-pans-pandas/

University of Minnesota Libraries Publishing edition, 2015. This edition adapted from a work originally produced in 2010 by a publisher who has requested that it not receive attribution. (2015, October 27). *2.3 personality and values*. Principles of Management. Retrieved March 28, 2023, from https://granite.pressbooks.pub/principlesmanagement/chapter/2-3-personality-and-values-3/

VAK test: What is your visual, auditory, and kinesthetic type? ProProfs. (n.d.). Retrieved March 28, 2023, from https://www.proprofs.com/quiz-school/story.php?title=vak-quiz-visual- auditory-kinesthetic

Valinsky, J. (2023, June 15). *Bud Light loses its title as America's top-selling beer | CNN business*. CNN. https://www.cnn.com/2023/06/14/business/bud-light-modelo-top-selling-may-sales/index.html

Valuer.ai. (2022, July 28). *50 brands that failed to innovate*. Valuer. https://www.valuer.ai/blog/50-examples-of-corporations-that-failed-to-innovate-and-missed-their-chance

Wauthia, E., Lefebvre, L., Huet, K., Blekic, W., El Bouragui, K., & Rossignol, M. (2019).

Weber, D. O. (2019, February 11). How many patients can a primary care physician treat?: AAPL publication. American Association for Physician Leadership - Inspiring Change.

World Health Organization. (2023, March 29). *Autism*. World Health Organization. https://www.who.int/news-room/fact-sheets/detail/autism-spectrum-disorders

WWT. (n.d.). https://www.wwt.com/

YouTube. (2012, October 19). Eric Ries explains the pivot. YouTube. Retrieved March 28, 2023, from https://www.youtube.com/watch?v=1hTI4z2ijc4

Zauderer, S. (2023, September 19). *PTSD vs. autism: Differences & similarities*. Life-Changing ABA Therapy - Cross River Therapy. https://www.crossrivertherapy.com/autism/ptsd-vs-autism#:

Made in the USA
Middletown, DE
09 November 2023